80 RECIPES MADE with chicken

For your slow Cooker

Chris Moore

Copyright © 2024 by Chris Moore
All rights reserved.

No portion of this book may be reproduced in any form without written permission from the publisher or author.

Table of Contents

- Best Chicken Formulas 1
- Simple Moroccan Chicken Sticks 1
- Simple Chicken Fajitas Bowls 2
- Chicken Schnitzel with Velvety Kale 5
- Ginger Scallion Chicken Bowls 8
- Simple Chicken Milanese 9
- Rich Tuscan Chicken Pasta 11
- Chicken Tawook Quinoa Bowls 13
- Greek Chicken and Potatoes 16
- Chicken Sticks with Cilantro Mint Sauce 18
- Cauliflower Rice Chicken Burrito Bowls 19
- Idiot proof Chicken Breasts 21
- Chicken Fajita Cobb Serving of mixed greens 22
- McCarthy Chopped Serving of mixed greens 24
- Summer Barbecued Chicken Control Serving of mixed greens 25
- Chicken Shawarma Bowls 27
- Flame broiled Chicken Panzanella 29
- Pesto Farmers Showcase Serving of mixed greens with Flame broiled Chicken 31
- Greek Chicken Serving of mixed greens 32
- Flame broiled Chicken with Avocado Tomato Serving of mixed greens 35
- Chicken Parmesan 36
- Chicken Parmesan Meatballs 37
- Chicken Parmesan Gnocchi Prepare 39
- Spaghetti Squash Chicken Parmesan Bake 40
- Mushroom Chicken Parmesan Pasta 41
- Chicken Parmesan Pizza 43
- Chicken Parmesan Panini 44

- Corny Chicken and Rice Casserole 47
- Asian Chicken Slaw 48
- Easy Chicken Pot Pie 49
- BBQ Chicken Quinoa Serving of mixed greens 51
- Barbecued BBQ Chicken Pizza 52
- Ginger Scallion Chicken Wraps 54
- Poblano Chicken Enchiladas 55
- Thai Chicken Pizza 57
- Custom made Chicken Taquitos 59
- Greek Chicken Stuffed Pitas 60
- Green Chicken Enchiladas 61
- Tex Mex Enchilada Queso 64
- Firm Chicken Thighs with Crushed Peas 65
- Butter Chicken 67
- Cuban Mojo Chicken Thighs 68
- Thai Chicken Coconut Curry 70
- Chipotle Chicken Lettuce Wraps 71
- Chicken Shish Kabobs 73
- Flame broiled Korean Chicken Sticks 74
- Lemon Chicken Pasta 75
- Shredded BBQ Chicken Burgers 76
- Hand crafted Orange Chicken 77
- Artichoke Pepper Braised Chicken 79
- Fresh Lemon Chicken Thighs 80
- Mushroom Chicken Marsala Pasta 82
- Brown Butter Chicken Pasta 83
- Chicken Paprikash 84
- Chicken Tagine with Olives 86

Simple Mexican Destroyed Chicken {Verde!} 88
Italian Wedding Soup 89
Simple White Chicken Chili 91
Chicken Tortilla Soup 92
Chicken Chili Verde...95
Stacked Chicken Pho (Instant Pot + Stove Best) 96
Smoky Chipotle Chicken Chili 99
Chicken Posole 100
Simple Mexican Shredded Chicken 102
Skillet Chipotle Chicken Enchilada Prepare 104
Green Chicken Enchiladas 105
DIY Chipotle Burrito Bowl 107
Simple Taco Serving of mixed greens 109
Ground Chicken Tacos 110
Chicken Tinga Tacos...112
Chrissy's Chicken Nachos with Avocado Salsa 114
Poblano Chicken Fajitas 116
Enfrijoladas 117
Tacky Chicken Taco Chili Pasta 118
Zuni Simmered Entire Chicken with Chimichurri 119
Flame broiled Lemonade Chicken 121
Lemon Broiled Spatchcock Chicken 123
Chicken Larb Bowls...124
Chicken Kofta Kebabs 126

Best Chicken Formulas

It's difficult figuring out what's for supper each night, but these chicken formulas are all beyond any doubt to be swarm pleasers. There's something for everybody here, from chicken breast formulas to chicken thigh formulas to 7 distinctive turns on chicken parmesan. Whether you're searching for a simple, speedy, or sound supper formula that can nourish your whole family or take off you with scraps for lunch, I've got a plenty of tasty chicken formulas that'll provide you a few thoughts of what to cook for supper.

Simple Moroccan Chicken Sticks

Our trip to Morocco and these Moroccan Chicken Sticks have been on my intellect as of late and I'm prepared to re-live that madly unimaginable get-away through a few of the flavor recollections I brought domestic like this Moroccan Tomato Serving of mixed greens and this Herbed Couscous!

Fixings & Substitutions

- Pulverized Ruddy Pepper
- Ground Turmeric
- Greek Yogurt
- Extra-Virgin Olive Oil
- Ruddy Wine Vinegar
- Tomato Glue
- Legitimate Salt
- Dark Pepper
- Garlic

- Lemons
- Boneless Skinless Chicken Thighs and/or Breasts
- Warm Pita Bread
- Additional Greek Yogurt
- Chopped Tomatoes
- New Mint

How to Create Moroccan Chicken Sticks

Step 1: Combine the smashed ruddy pepper and ground turmeric in expansive bowl and blend in 2 tablespoons of hot water and let stand for 5 minutes.

Step 2: Include the Greek yogurt, olive oil, ruddy wine vinegar, tomato glue, 2 teaspoons salt, and 1 teaspoon dark pepper to zest blend in bowl; whisk to combine.

Step 3: Mix in garlic and lemon juice.

Step 4: Include the chicken. Cover and chill for AT Slightest 1 hour. I do for 4 least and yes you'll do overnight in the event that you incline toward

Step 5: Get ready the barbecue over medium-high warm. String chicken pieces on sticks, partitioning similarly. Dispose of marinade in bowl. Sprinkle each stick with salt and pepper.

Step 6: Barbecue chicken until brilliant brown and cooked through, turning sticks sometimes, 10 to 12 minutes add up to. Exchange sticks to platter. Serve with serving recommendations and additional lemon wedges

Simple Chicken Fajitas Bowls

I'll eat fajitas every what direction whether it's chicken fajitas, steak fajitas, shrimp fajitas, fajita quesadillas... you title it. I will moreover eat bowls for lunch regular of the week. Case in point this make at domestic Chipotle Burrito Bowl that is on repeat week after week.

Chicken Fajitas Bowl Fixings

Chicken Breasts - cut into lean strips and after that marinated for an hour

Marinade - lime juice, olive oil, minced garlic, salt, ground cumin, chili powder, and ruddy pepper drops

Peppers - a blend of poblano peppers and chime peppers

Onions - we're utilizing ruddy and yellow here

Rice - for the foundation of the bowl

Fixings - dark beans, charred corn, tomatoes, guacamole, lime, and cilantro

Step by Step

Within the foot of a zip beat pack or bowl combine the marinade fixings, lime juice, olive oil, garlic, salt, cumin, chili powder and ruddy pepper drops and whisk to combine. Another meagerly cut the chicken breasts into strips, approximately the estimate of your finger. Add the chicken in, blend until it's equitably coated within the marinade, pop it within the cooler and let marinate for 1 hour.

When you're prepared to cook the Chicken Fajitas warm a huge cast press skillet over tall warm. Include a tablespoon of olive oil. Include the chicken blend, marinade included, and sauté until fully cooked. Employing a combine of tongs, evacuate the chicken from the skillet and include the vegetables. Sauté until tender and charred. Include the chicken back into the cast press skillet and hurl to combine.

Serve the Chicken Fajitas in a bowl with rice, dark beans, charred corn, chopped tomatoes, a huge spoonful of guacamole, cilantro, and a wedge of lime.

Varieties and Substitutions

Chicken Breasts - feel free to utilize chicken thighs in the event that you lean toward both work awesome in this formula

Poblano Peppers - in the event that you're serving Chicken Fajitas for kids feel free to utilize more chime peppers instep

Rice - white rice, earthy colored rice, or cauliflower rice will work

Dark Beans - feel free to substitute for pinto beans if that's what you favor or all you've got on hand

Charred Corn - I purchase my charred corn solidified from Dealer Joes but you'll moreover char a cob of corn yourself

Garnishes - utilize your favorites here. Destroyed cheese, acrid cream, and salsa would moreover be scrumptious augmentations.

For the Chicken
- 1 ½ pounds Chicken Breasts
- 2 tablespoons lime juice
- 3 tablespoons olive oil
- 3 cloves garlic, minced
- ½ teaspoon salt
- ½ teaspoon Ground Cumin
- ½ teaspoon Chili Powder
- ½ teaspoon Red Pepper Chips
- For the veggies
- 1 poblano pepper daintily cut
- 1 ruddy chime pepper meagerly cut
- 1 yellow pepper daintily cut
- ½ yellow onion meagerly cut
- ½ ruddy onion daintily cut
- For the Bowls
- 3 mugs steamed white rice
- 1 container dark beans, flushed and depleted
- 1 container Charred Corn

- 1 container Chopped Tomatoes
- 1 recipe Guacamole
- Limes
- Fresh Cilantro

Enlightening

Cut the chicken breasts into lean strips, almost the measure of your finger. Combine the lime juice, olive oil, garlic, salt, cumin, chili powder and ruddy pepper flakes in a bowl and whisk to combine. Include the chicken and marinate for 1 hour.

Warm an expansive cast press skillet over high warm. Include a tablespoon of olive oil. Include the chicken blend, marinade included, and sauté until completely cooked. Employing a match of tongs, expel the chicken from the skillet and add the vegetables. Sauté until delicate and charred. Include the chicken back into the cast press skillet and hurl to combine.

Serve in a bowl with rice, dull beans, singed corn, cleaved tomatoes, a huge spoonful of guacamole and a wedge of lime.

Chicken Schnitzel with Velvety Kale

To begin with things to begin with - what is schnitzel. On the off chance that you've never listened of it sometime recently - it's a lean cut of meat that's ordinarily breaded and after that fricasseed in fat. More times than not, in the event that you're in Europe, it's pork based. But in my family we did it 10 times outta 10 with chicken and browned it in a few olive oil. Keeping it light over here within the Dalkin clan

Fixings

- 4 4-6 ounce skinless boneless chicken bosoms
- Genuine salt and freshly ground dim pepper

- 1 glass all-purpose flour
- 1 lemon, zested
- 1 teaspoon garlic powder
- 2 huge eggs
- 2 mugs panko breadcrumbs
- 4 tablespoons olive oil
- Freshly chopped chives
- Lemon wedges

For the Rich Kale

- 2 lbs kale, (generally 3 bunches), stems evacuated and clears out generally chopped into 1 inch pieces
- ½ glass olive oil
- Kosher salt and naturally broken dark pepper
- 1 lemon, zested and juiced
- 2 ounces cream cheddar, at room temp
- 2 ounces ground fontina cheese
- ⅓ glass overwhelming cream

Informational

For the Chicken Schnitzel

- Put the chicken breasts in a plastic sack, one at a time, and pound them so they are approximately ½ inch thick all through its aggregate.
- Plan 3 bowls, one with flour, salt, pepper, lemon pizzazz and the garlic powder, one with whisked eggs and the final with Panko bread pieces.
- Put each piece of chicken within the flour, coating both sides, and shaking off any overabundance. Another dunk it into the whisked egg

- let any overabundance fluid deplete off. Another, coat it with the Panko breadcrumbs.
- Put a huge skillet over medium tall warm and include the olive oil. When the oil is hot, painstakingly put one piece of Chicken Schnitzel into the holder and let it cook for 3-5 minutes and after that flip it over to wrap up cooking. Each piece ought to be brilliant brown on both sides.
- Evacuate the chicken to a paper towel lined plate and rehash the method with the remaining chicken. Once all the chicken is cooked, grant it all a liberal press of lemon and an expansive spoonful of the velvety kale. Alter salt and pepper to taste.

For the Velvety Kale
- In a huge bowl, include the kale and ¼ container of olive oil and season with salt. Massage the kale to tenderize for 2-3 minutes. The kale ought to begin to shrivel and shrivel.
- Warm the remaining olive oil in your biggest pot or Dutch broiler. Include the kale in clumps, blending to shrink indeed encourage until all the kale has been included. Cover the pot and cook on medium-low, blending each few minutes, until the kale is delicate, approximately 30 minutes. In case the kale begins to brown, diminish warm to moo and proceed to cook. Mix within the lemon pizzazz and lemon juice and expel from the warm.
- Break the cream cheese into little pieces and drop them into the Dutch stove with the kale, whereas still over moo warm. Mix the cream cheese until it's completely combined into the kale. Include the fontina and overwhelming cream and combine for around 1 minute until the fontina is dissolved.

Ginger Scallion Chicken Bowls

These bowls are great for anyone trying to find a straightforward weeknight supper that still looks favor sufficient to serve visitors. Also, they're pressed with parts of nutritious fixings like chicken, vegetables, and flavor-packed ginger and scallion sauce—so you'll feel good about bolstering them (and yourself!) delightful nourishment. Prepared for takeoff? Let's get begun on making these mind blowing Ginger Scallion Chicken Bowls!

Fixings & Substitutions

- ½ head napa cabbage destroyed
- ½ head purple cabbage destroyed
- 1 yellow ringer pepper cut into matchsticks
- 1 ruddy chime pepper cut into matchsticks
- 6 ounces shitake mushrooms cut
- 2 tablespoons vegetable oil
- 2 cooked chicken breasts destroyed

For the Ginger/Scallion sauce:

- 1 bunch scallions meagerly cut (around 1 ¼ glass add up to)
- 1 3- inch piece of ginger peeled and exceptionally finely minced
- 4 cloves garlic minced
- 4 teaspoons toasted sesame oil
- 8 tablespoons soy sauce
- 4 tablespoons rice vinegar
- ⅓ container vegetable oil
- 1 teaspoon ruddy pepper pieces
- Fixings
- 1 english cucumber sliced
- 3 glasses cooked white rice
- 1-2 tablespoons rice wine vinegar

- 2 avocados thinly sliced
- 2-3 glasses meagerly destroyed romaine lettuce

How to Create Ginger Scallion Chicken Bowls

Step 1: In an expansive bowl combine the napa cabbage, purple cabbage, yellow and ruddy bell pepper.

Step 2: In a medium skillet, saute the mushrooms within the oil until brilliant brown, approximately 8-10 minutes.

Step 3: Once golden, remove and include to the cabbage mixture at the side the destroyed chicken breasts.

Step 4: Combine the fixings for the Ginger Scallion sauce in a bowl.

Step 5: Put half of the sauce aside to utilize for sprinkling, and combine the remaining half with the cabbage and chicken blend and hurl to combine.

Step 6: Prep the toppings, sliced cucumber, steamed white rice hurled with 1-2 tablespoons of rice wine vinegar, cut avocados and romaine lettuce.

Step 7: Prep the garnishes, cut cucumber, steamed white rice hurled with 1-2 tablespoons of rice wine vinegar, cut avocados and romaine lettuce.

Simple Chicken Milanese

In case you've never listened of Chicken Milanese some time recently – it's a chicken cutlet that's beat lean, breaded in Panko bread pieces, and after that fricasseed in olive oil. The result could be a super firm, delicious, and flavorful piece of chicken. It's essentially a celebrated Chicken Piece and I'm fixated!

I like to serve Chicken Milanese with an enormous green serving of mixed greens like this Butter Lettuce Serving of mixed greens or this Arugula Pesto & White Bean Panzanella. A German Potato Serving of mixed greens or The Finest Mascarpone Squashed Potatoes would too be delightful.

Furthermore, maybe a couple of Silly Creamed Kale or Cooked Broccolini with Lemon and Garlic to round everything out.

How to Cook Chicken Milanese

Step 1: Put the chicken breasts in a plastic sack, one at a time, and pound them so they are almost ⅓ inch thick all through its aggregate. Think super lean and Expansive. So it takes up a entirety supper plate.

I utilize a meat hammer or wooden rolling to pound the chicken, but in case you do not have either, you'll utilize an overwhelming foot pot or container.

Stage 2: Plan 3 dishes, one with flour, salt, pepper, lemon outfit and-go and the garlic powder, one with whisked eggs and the last with Panko bread pieces mixed with parmesan cheddar.

Step 3: Put each piece of chicken within the flour, coating both sides, and shaking off any overabundance.

Step 4: Following dunk it into the whisked egg – let any overabundance fluid deplete off.

Step 5: Another, coat it with the Panko breadcrumbs cheese mixture.

Step 6: Put a huge skillet over medium tall warm and include the olive oil. Once the oil is hot, carefully put one piece of chicken into the container and let it cook for 3-5 minutes and after that flip it over to wrap up cooking. Each piece ought to be brilliant brown on both sides.

Step 7: Expel the chicken to a paper towel lined plate and rehash the method with the remaining chicken. Once all the chicken is cooked, give it all a liberal crush of lemon, a sprinkle of the upland cress, and season with more salt as required.

- 2 4-6 ounce skinless boneless chicken breasts
- Legitimate salt and newly ground dark pepper
- ½ container all-purpose flour
- 1 lemon zested
- 1 teaspoon garlic powder

- 2 large eggs
- 1 container panko breadcrumbs
- 1 container new parmesan cheese finely ground
- 4 tablespoons olive oil
- 1-2 bunches upland cress hurled with olive oil, lemon juice, salt and pepper
- lemon wedges

Rich Tuscan Chicken Pasta

Rich Tuscan Chicken Pasta was another of my experience growing up favs adjacent to that Garlic Buttered Favored courier Hair from numerous weeks back. The creamy tomato sauce made with both canned tomatoes and sun dried tomatoes is brilliant. And makes the culminate sauce for a few pasta to swim within. The chicken is essential and simply adds a touch of protein. In case you need to amp it up, and utilize a darkened chicken formula, utilize the zest rub from here. It unquestionably seasons things up a little and that is not persistently everybody's stick.

Fixings
- 1 pound spaghetti or linguini
- 2 tablespoons olive oil
- 1 pound boneless skinless chicken breasts
- Kosher salt and crisply split dark pepper to taste
- 4 cuts bacon
- 8 cloves garlic, roughly chopped
- 1 15-ounce can canned diced tomatoes
- ½ cup sun dried tomatoes, generally chopped
- 1 modest bunch infant spinach

- ½ container overwhelming cream
- ½ - 1 glass crisply ground parmesan cheese
- 1 lemon, zested and juiced
- basil to embellish

Enlightening

- Cook the pasta until al dente. Save 1 cup of pasta water once cooked, deplete and set aside.
- Warm a huge skillet over medium-high warm with the olive oil. Generously season the chicken with salt and pepper and cook until brilliant on the outside and now not pink interior, approximately 7-8 minutes per side. Evacuate from the container, let rest for 10 minutes before thinly cutting.
- Within the same skillet, include the bacon and cook until crispy. Drain on a paper towel lined plate and after that tear into nibble measured pieces.
- In case there's a parcel of bacon fat remaining, deplete most of it off. Include the garlic, tomatoes, sun dried tomatoes and spinach to the skillet and cook over medium warm until fragrant, around 2 minutes. Season with salt and pepper to taste, then add overwhelming cream, Parmesan, and some tablespoons of saved pasta water. Simmer for 5 minutes until impudent and combined.
- Include the saved pasta, chicken, bacon, lemon juice and lemon get-up-and-go and hurl until combined. On the off chance that it's as well thick, include some more tablespoons of the saved pasta water. Decorate with basil and serve.

Chicken Tawook Quinoa Bowls

It's as simple as including a few barbecued chicken breast sticks on best of a quinoa bowl, hummus, garlic sauce, avocados, cucumbers and a bit of shredded lettuce and lunch or supper is DONE!

For the Chicken:
- ¼ glass lemon juice
- ¼ container vegetable oil
- ¾ container plain yogurt
- 4 cloves garlic finely chopped
- 2 teaspoons tomato glue
- 2 teaspoons red wine vinegar
- 1 ½ teaspoons salt
- 1 teaspoon dried oregano
- ¼ teaspoon paprika
- ¼ teaspoon ground dark pepper
- ¼ teaspoon ground allspice
- 2 pounds skinless boneless chicken breast parts - cut into 2 inch pieces
- fresh parsley

For the Bowls:
- 2 mugs cooked quinoa
- 2 ready avocado
- ½ cup hand crafted Hummus
- store bought garlic sauce
- sliced Persian cucumbers
- 1 head romaine lettuce destroyed
- served w/a side of pita bread
- ½ glass hand crafted Tzatziki discretionary

Enlightening
- Whisk together the lemon juice, vegetable oil, plain yogurt, garlic, tomato glue, salt, oregano, paprika, pepper and allspice in a huge bowl; include the chicken and hurl to coat. Transfer the chicken blend into a huge plastic bag; refrigerate at slightest 4 hours.
- Preheat an indoor or open air barbecue for medium-high warm and delicately oil grind. String the chicken onto metal or wooden sticks. Cook on preheated grill until the chicken is golden and now not pink within the center, almost 5 minutes each side. Sprinkle the parsley over the sticks.
- To gather, isolate the quinoa into 4 bowls and top with rise to parts of avocado, hummus, garlic sauce, sliced cucumbers and destroyed lettuce. Season with salt, pepper and lemon juice in the event that required. Serve promptly.

Chicken Caesar Serving of mixed greens Pizza
Fixings
- 1 lb pizza batter
- Olive oil for brushing outside
- 2 cloves garlic cut
- 8 ounces mozzarella cut
- ½ container ground Parmesan additionally little chunk for shaving
- 1 chicken breast flame broiled and cut daintily
- 2 romaine hearts washed and dried, cut into ½-inch pieces
- ½ container Caesar Serving of mixed greens Dressing formula takes after
- Caesar Serving of mixed greens Dressing:

- Fit salt and freshly broken dim pepper
- ½ glass ground Parmesan
- ⅓ glass mayonnaise
- ¼ container lemon juice
- 2 tablespoons olive oil
- 2 teaspoons Dijon mustard
- 1 teaspoon Worcestershire sauce
- 1 teaspoon legitimate salt
- ½ teaspoon naturally split dark pepper
- 2 cloves garlic minced or ground

Informational

- Get ready a gas or charcoal barbecue to tall warm. Brush the barbecue with a bit of oil. Whereas the barbecue is getting warm, make the Caesar Dressing. In a blender or sustenance processor, set up the Parmesan, mayonnaise, lemon juice, olive oil, mustard, Worcestershire, salt, pepper and garlic until emulsified and smooth. Refrigerate until prepared to utilize.
- Shape the batter into 2 medium-ish pizzas whereas on a clean floured surface. Let the batter sit for 5 minutes and after that re-form to create beyond any doubt it's as huge as you'd like. Put the pizza batter on a delicately floured rimless heating sheet, or pizza peel. Exchange the batter over to the barbecue, and slide the pizza batter specifically onto the barbecue. Barbecue the dough for almost 2 minutes with the top closed. Employing a match of tongs, lift the top, and flip the batter over onto the other side and cook for almost 2 minutes more. The batter ought to be brilliant brown with flame broil marks on both sides.

- Brush the olive oil over the pizza and sprinkle with garlic. Once the mixture is cooked, expel it from the barbecue and put it back onto the heating sheet.
- Orchestrate the mozzarella, parmesan and chicken breast cuts on beat. and put back onto the flame broil until the cheese has softened. Utilizing tongs, evacuate the pizza from the barbecue and beat with the dressed romaine takes off and season with salt and pepper as required. Decorate with long strips of parmesan cheese. Cut and serve instantly.

Greek Chicken and Potatoes

Greek Chicken and Potatoes is one of those comforting one-skillet suppers that takes care of trade on bleak winter days.

Everything gets heaped into an enormous cast press skillet, prepared with a marinade so addicting you'll need to drink it, and broiled until the chicken and the potatoes are brilliant, fresh and immaculate flawlessness!

Fixings
- ½ container new lemon juice
- 4 cloves garlic generally chopped
- 4 tablespoons new flat-leaf parsley finely chopped
- 2 tablespoons basil finely chopped
- 1 tablespoon new oregano finely chopped
- 1 tablespoon rosemary finely chopped
- 1 tablespoon thyme finely chopped
- 1 teaspoon ruddy pepper chips
- ½ container olive oil

- 1 entire chicken cut down into breasts, thighs and legs
- 6 medium Yukon Gold Potatoes cut into nibble measured pieces
- Legitimate salt and freshly broken dull pepper

Discretionary Garnishes

- Cucumber medium dice
- Cherry Tomatoes divided
- Crumbled Feta

Informational

- Mix together the lemon juice, garlic, herbs, ruddy pepper pieces and olive oil in a bowl. Put the chicken in an expansive zip bolt pack and pour ¾th of the marinade on best. Marinate within the cooler for 12-24 hours.
- Once the chicken is marinated, preheat stove to 375 degrees F.
- Put the potatoes in a huge bowl and sprinkle with the remaining marinade, hurl to combine. Season the potatoes with salt and pepper. Orchestrate the potatoes on the foot of a huge cast press skillet. Evacuate the chicken from the marinade and put on best of the potatoes and season the chicken with salt and pepper.
- Broil the chicken and potatoes within the stove for 1 hour 15 minutes until brilliant and fresh.
- Best with the chopped cucumbers, cherry tomatoes and feta and serve quickly.

NOTES

Be beyond any doubt that the pieces of chicken might cook at distinctive rates. A thermometer is your best wagered here!

Chicken Sticks with Cilantro Mint Sauce

Chicken breast marinated in a greek yogurt blend, at that point barbecued until just slightly charred on the exterior. Dunk it within the cilantro mint sauce and/or tzatziki! The more plunges the superior!

Fixings

For the Chicken Sticks:

- ¼ glass lemon juice
- ¼ glass vegetable oil
- ¾ glass plain greek yogurt
- 4 cloves garlic finely chopped
- 2 teaspoons tomato glue
- 2 teaspoons ruddy wine vinegar
- 1 ½ teaspoons salt
- 1 teaspoon dried oregano
- ¼ teaspoon paprika
- ¼ teaspoon ground dark pepper
- ¼ teaspoon ground allspice
- 2 pounds skinless boneless chicken bosoms - cut into 2 inch pieces

For the Cilantro Mint Sauce:

- 2 glasses pressed new cilantro
- 1 container pressed new mint takes off
- 1 shallot
- ¼ container water
- 1 tablespoon new lime juice
- 1 teaspoon chopped serrano pepper
- 1 teaspoon sugar
- kosher salt and naturally split pepper to taste

Additional:

- Pita wedges optional
- Tzatziki discretionary

Informational

- Whisk together the lemon juice, vegetable oil, plain yogurt, garlic, tomato glue, salt, oregano, paprika, pepper and allspice in an expansive bowl; include the chicken and hurl to coat. Exchange the chicken blend into a huge plastic pack; refrigerate at slightest 4 hours.
- Preheat an indoor or open air barbecue for medium-high warm and delicately oil grind. String the chicken onto metal or wooden sticks. Cook on preheated flame broil until the chicken is brilliant and now not pink in the center, approximately 5 minutes each side.
- Combine the fixings for the mint cilantro sauce in a blender and mix until smooth. Alter salt and pepper as required.
- Serve the chicken sticks with the cilantro and mint sauce and pita and a raita

NOTES

The cilantro mint sauce would moreover be awesome on steak or salmon.

Cauliflower Rice Chicken Burrito Bowls

This burrito bowl is stacked with a chipotle marinated chicken, bounty of beans, corn, pico, avocado and a sprinkling of cheese for great degree.

Fixings

For the Chicken

- 1 tablespoon vegetable oil
- 2 chipotle peppers in adobo finely slashed

- 1 teaspoon garlic powder
- 1 teaspoon ground cumin
- ½ teaspoon dried oregano
- ½ teaspoon dark pepper
- 4 boneless skinless chicken thighs (or 3 boneless, skinless chicken bosoms)

For the Bowls
- 3 mugs cauliflower florets
- 1 glass cooked dark beans depleted and flushed
- 1 cup charred corn
- 1 avocado cut or cubed
- ½ glass chopped cilantro
- 1 lime cut into wedges
- olive oil
- sea salt and naturally ground dark pepper
- Crema
- Pico de Gallo
- Shredded Monterey Jack

Informational
- Combine the vegetable oil, chopped chipotle peppers in adobo, garlic powder, cumin, dried oregano, and dark pepper in a little bowl and mix to combine. Put the chicken in a huge zip best plastic pack and include the marinade. Zip the sack and mix the chicken into the marinade. Put it into the ice chest and let it marinate for at slightest 1 hour.
- Warm an indoor or open air barbecue to approximately 400 degrees F (medium tall warm). Put the chicken onto the flame broil and flame broil 5 to 6 minutes per side, until the chicken is cooked. Evacuate

the chicken from the grill and let rest for 10 minutes. Chop the chicken into little chomp measured pieces and utilize as required.

- Make beyond any doubt your cauliflower is completely dry. Put the cauliflower in a nourishment processor and beat until it has the surface of rice. Work in bunches in case essential and do not over prepare or it will get soft. In a huge skillet, warm 1 teaspoon of olive oil over medium warm. Include the cauliflower and sauté until warmed through, almost 5 minutes. Season with salt, pepper and a crush of lime juice to assist expel any sharpness from the crude cauliflower. Evacuate from the skillet and parcel the "rice" into 4 serving bowls.
- To the bowls include the chicken, dark beans, charred corn, avocado, and cilantro, pico, cheese and serve with limes.

NOTES

Feel free to swap out proteins! Too in case you appreciate rice, by all means utilize that rather than cauliflower or go halfsies.

Idiot proof Chicken Breasts

This recipe for Secure Chicken Breasts is going to create all our lives interminably way better.

Fixings

- 2 8 to 10-ounce boneless, skin on chicken breasts (I continuously inquire my butcher for bone in - skin on chicken breasts and inquire that the expel the bone for me)
- 2-3 tablespoons Gaby's Go To Flavoring
- Salt and naturally ground dark pepper
- 2 tablespoons olive oil

Enlightening
- Cover the breasts with plastic wrap and pound the thick portion tenderly with a meat pounder, rolling stick, or an overwhelming skillet until the chicken is an indeed ⅔-inch thickness.
- Pat each chicken breast dry with paper towels and sprinkle each breast with legitimate salt, crisply broken black pepper and equal amounts of Gaby's Go To Flavoring.
- Pour the oil in a 12-inch skillet (ideally cast-iron) and warm over medium tall warm. Include the chicken and cook until the side confronting down starts to turn brilliant brown and the meat starts to turn misty along the edges, 5 to 7 minutes. In case you attempt to turn the chicken and it feels stuck, it isn't brilliant and firm or prepared to flip.
- Flip the chicken and proceed to cook the chicken over medium warm until the skin is well browned and fresh, 5 to 7 minutes. Exchange a sautéed chicken breast to each plate and let rest a few minutes earlier to cutting and serving.

Chicken Fajita Cobb Serving of mixed greens
Fixings:
- Boneless Skinless Chicken Thighs – Feel free to substitute for chicken breasts.
- Vegetable Oil
- Chipotle Peppers in Adobo
- Garlic Powder
- Ground Cumin

- Dried Oregano
- Legitimate Salt
- Dark Pepper
- Showcase Greens
- Corn on the Cob
- Cherry Tomatoes
- Chime Peppers
- Avocados
- Feta
- Lemon
- Garlic
- Shallot
- Ruddy Wine Vinegar
- Olive Oil

How to Form Chicken Fajita Cobb Serving of mixed greens

Stage 1: Consolidate the vegetable oil, hacked chipotle peppers in adobo, garlic powder, cumin, dried oregano, salt and dull pepper in a little bowl and mix to join.

Step 2: Put the chicken in an expansive zip beat plastic pack and include the marinade. Zip the sack and mix the chicken into the marinade. Put it into the ice chest and let it marinate for at slightest 1 hour.

Step 3: Warm an indoor or outdoor grill to approximately 400 degrees F (medium tall warm). Put the chicken onto the flame broil and barbecue 5 to 6 minutes per side, until the chicken is cooked.

Step 4: Expel the chicken from the flame broil and let rest for 10 minutes. Cut the chicken against the grain and utilize as needed.

Step 5: On an expansive platter organize the greens with all the fixings on beat. Whisk the fixings for the vinaigrette together. Hurl the serving of mixed greens with the vinaigrette and serve.

How to Store Chicken Fajita Cobb Serving of mixed greens

This is often best eaten fresh. It would be best to make as much as you would like and you'll be able continuously store additional chicken in an hermetically sealed holder within the fridge for 3-4 days. In any case, the serving of mixed greens ought to ideally be amassed new. You'll also store any extra vinaigrette within the cooler for a few days.

How to Solidify Chicken Fajita Cobb Serving of mixed greens

You'll solidify any remaining chicken in the cooler for 3 months. As with storage, rest of the serving of mixed greens fixings ought to be collected new. Fair defrost the chicken some time recently eating and appropriately warm it through when it's time to eat.

McCarthy Chopped Serving of mixed greens
Fixings
For the Serving of mixed greens:
- 2 glasses romaine chopped
- ½ glass barbecued chicken diced
- ¼ container child cherry tomatoes split
- ½ container ruddy beets diced (completely permitted to purchase them pre-roasted at TJ's, Entirety Nourishments etc.)
- ½ container cucumbers diced
- ½ container chickpeas
- ¼ glass bacon diced
- ¼ glass sharp cheddar cheese diced

- 1 avocado diced
- Kosher salt and crisply broken dark pepper to taste

For the Dressing:
- 3 tablespoons olive oil
- 1 tablespoon ruddy wine vinegar
- 1 tablespoon new lemon juice
- 1 clove garlic simmered
- Kosher salt and naturally broken dark pepper to taste

Enlightening

For the Serving of mixed greens:
- Chop everything, make it into a beautiful serving of mixed greens, and serve.

For the Dressing:
- For the dressing, whisk everything together to combine, breaking up the broiled clove of garlic so it's equally joined.

NOTES

There are two ways to serve this - as of now chopped, or lined up like a rainbow on a huge platter.

Summer Barbecued Chicken Control Serving of mixed greens

Summer Flame broiled Chicken Control Serving of mixed greens with sweet blueberries, disintegrated bacon and a lemon vinaigrette is the serving of mixed greens of summer!

Fixings

For the Serving of mixed greens
- 4 cuts thick cut bacon

- 1 half quart blueberries
- ¼ glass disintegrated goat or feta cheese
- 1 modest bunch little basil takes off
- 4 mugs ranchers advertise lettuce
- 2 corn on the cob bits expelled
- 1-2 avocados

For the Chicken

- ½ pound boneless skinless chicken breasts
- Kosher salt and crisply broken dark pepper
- 1 tablespoon olive oil
- 1 tablespoon chopped new rosemary
- 1 tablespoon chopped new thyme
- 1 tablespoons dried oregano

For the Lemon Champagne vinaigrette

- 2 garlic cloves finely chopped
- 1 tablespoon Dijon Mustard
- ¼ container champagne vinegar
- 2 tablespoons new lemon juice
- 2 tablespoons nectar
- 1 teaspoon ruddy pepper chips
- ½ teaspoon salt
- ½ teaspoon crisply ground dark pepper
- ½ container additional virgin olive oil

Enlightening

- Warm a huge cast press skillet over medium warm and include the bacon. Cook until new and the fat is delivered. Expel the bacon and exchange it on a paper towel lined plate. Deplete off most of the bacon oil, clearing out around 2 teaspoons.

- Season the chicken with salt and pepper and coat with the new and dried spices. Within the same skillet, over medium-high warm, include the chicken to bacon oil and cook until brilliant and fresh on both sides, around 5 to 6 minutes per side. Evacuate the chicken and let rest. Cut into pieces when prepared to serve.
- In a huge bowl, collect the serving of mixed greens. Begin with the bed of lettuce, include the chicken, blueberries, cheese, basil takes off, torn up bacon, avocado and corn. Sprinkle with the vinaigrette. Serve instantly.

For the vinaigrette
- Combine all the fixings and whisk together. Taste and alter salt and pepper as required.

NOTES

What could be a control serving of mixed greens? It has all the protein and fiber you would like to keep controlling through your day! Swap out the vinaigrette depending on what you've got on hand.

Chicken Shawarma Bowls

1000% completely fixated with this Chicken Shawarma formula!!

Fixings

For the Chicken
- 2 lemons juiced
- ½ container olive oil
- 6 cloves garlic stripped, squashed and minced
- Kosher salt and naturally split dark pepper
- 2 teaspoons ground cumin

- 2 teaspoons paprika
- ½ teaspoon dried oregano
- ½ teaspoon red-pepper chips
- 2 pounds boneless skinless chicken thighs

To Serve
- Romaine Lettuce destroyed
- Fluffy Pita Bread
- Olives

Informational
- In a gigantic zip-top pack, join the lemon juice, ½ glass olive oil, garlic, salt, pepper, cumin, paprika, oregano and red-pepper pieces. Include the chicken, zip the best of the sack and provide it a fast shake to combine. Fridge for at slightest 1 hour and up to 12 hours.
- Preheat a cast press to medium tall warm. Evacuate the chicken from the marinade and flame broil each chicken thigh for 4-5 minutes on each side until done. Expel and set aside to rest.
- Cut the chicken against the grain into lean strips and transfer back into the skillet and sauté for 2 minutes until fair somewhat firm around the edges.
- Exchange to a serving platter and serve with all the other parts of the supper party and accouterments.

NOTES

Keep more tzatziki on the side after you serve, and unquestionably make or purchase pita chips!

Flame broiled Chicken Panzanella

One of those main course servings of mixed greens that you'll need to appreciate all summer long!

Fixings

For the serving of mixed greens:

- 2 pounds colorful treasure tomatoes cut into wedges
- 1 half quart cherry tomatoes split
- 1 English cucumber split, cut into ½-inch half moons
- ½ little ruddy onion meagerly cut
- ½ container set castelvetrano olives split
- fresh basil to decorate

For the Chicken

- 1 pound chicken breasts
- 4 tablespoons olive oil
- 2 lemons pizzazz naturally ground and juiced
- 4 garlic cloves chopped
- 4 tablespoons new dill chopped
- 1 tablespoon ruddy wine vinegar
- Kosher salt and naturally split dark pepper
- 1 teaspoon smoked paprika
- ½ teaspoon cumin

For the Croutons:

- 1 9-ounce baguette cut
- 8 tablespoons olive oil
- 4 cloves garlic chopped
- 1 teaspoon Gaby's Go To flavoring

***For the Vinaigrette*:**

- 1 shallot generally chopped

- 2 cloves garlic chopped
- 1 lemon juiced
- 4 teaspoons champagne vinegar
- ⅓ glass olive oil
- kosher salt to taste

Informational

For the Chicken

- Combine the chicken with the marinade fixings and marinate for 2 hours. Once marinated, expel from the marinade, and flame broil both sides until fair cooked through. Exchange to cutting board and let rest 10 minutes. Cut against the grain and exchange to a huge serving bowl. Include the tomatoes, cherry tomatoes, cucumber, olives and ruddy onion. Include bread garnishes and dressing

For the Bread garnishes

- Sprinkle the bread with olive oil, garlic and flavoring blend. Exchange cut bread to barbecue. Barbecue for 5-7 minutes until each side is brilliant brown. Evacuate from flame broil and let cool some time recently tearing separated and serving. Include to serving of mixed greens fixings

For the Vinaigrette:

- Combine all the fixings and whisk until emulsified. Sprinkle over serving of mixed greens. Include basil as required.

To Assemble

- Combine all components on a huge platter and sprinkle with the vinaigrette. Toss and serve promptly.

NOTES

The vinaigrette endures for a week in the fridge, and I guarantee you'll need to slather it on everything! And the bread garnishes make a ton so I know you'll nibble on them as well.

Pesto Farmers Showcase Serving of mixed greens with Flame broiled Chicken

A stacked agriculturists advertise serving of mixed greens with all sorts of new deliver, bacon, some grilled chicken, and the foremost delish pesto vinaigrette.

Fixings

For the Serving of mixed greens:
- 4 cuts thick cut bacon
- 1 half quart blueberries
- 1 half quart little strawberries
- 1 sheet feta cubed
- 1 modest bunch little basil clears out
- Fresh chives
- 4 glasses ranchers showcase lettuce
- Medium legacy tomatoes cut
- 2 avocados meagerly cut

For the Chicken:
- ½ pound boneless skinless chicken breasts
- Kosher salt and naturally broken dark pepper
- 1 tablespoon olive oil
- 1 tablespoon chopped new rosemary
- 1 tablespoon chopped new thyme
- 1 tablespoons dried oregano

For the Pesto vinaigrette:
- 4 tablespoons Barilla Conventional Basil Pesto
- 2 tablespoons new lemon juice
- ½ glass additional virgin olive oil
- Kosher salt and naturally split dark pepper to taste

Informational
- Heat a expansive cast press skillet over medium warm and include the bacon. Cook until firm and the fat is rendered. Expel the bacon and exchange it on a paper towel lined plate. Drain off a large portion of the bacon oil, taking off around 2 teaspoons. Season the chicken with salt and pepper and coat with the new and dried herbs. Within the same skillet, over medium-high heat, include the chicken to bacon oil and cook until brilliant and fresh on both sides, around 5 to 6 minutes per side. Expel the chicken and let rest. Cut into pieces when prepared to serve.

For the vinaigrette:
- Combine the Barilla Pesto with the remaining fixings in a little bowl and whisk together. Taste and alter salt and pepper as required.
- Gathering:
- In an expansive bowl, collect the serving of mixed greens. Begin with the bed of lettuce, add the chicken, and after that everything else. Sprinkle with the vinaigrette. Serve immediately.

NOTES

The vinaigrette endures for a week in the fridge.

Greek Chicken Serving of mixed greens

It's like a bowl of the foremost mind blowing stuff on soil. Tart chicken, arugula, salted onions, feta cheese, cucumbers, tomatoes and a scrumptious lemon oregano vinaigrette.

Fixings

For the Chicken:
- 2 lemons juiced

- ½ container olive oil
- 6 cloves garlic stripped, squashed and minced
- 1 teaspoon legitimate salt
- 2 teaspoons crisply ground dark pepper
- 2 teaspoons ground cumin
- 2 teaspoons paprika
- ½ teaspoon dried oregano
- ½ teaspoon red-pepper pieces
- 2 pounds boneless skinless chicken thighs

For the Serving of mixed greens:
- 1-2 mugs new arugula
- Fresh parsley torn
- ½ container cherry tomatoes parts
- crumbled feta cheese
- ½ container cucumber split and meagerly cut
- pickled ruddy onions formula underneath

Lemon Oregano Vinaigrette
- 1 lemon juiced
- 2 teaspoons champagne vinegar
- ⅓ glass olive oil
- 2 cloves garlic minced
- ½ shallot minced
- kosher salt to taste
- fresh oregano

Salted red onions
- ½ mugs apple cider vinegar
- 1 tablespoon white sugar
- 1 ½ teaspoons legitimate salt

- 1 red onion daintily cut

Enlightening

- In a huge zip-top pack, join the lemon juice, ½ glass olive oil, garlic, salt, pepper, cumin, paprika, oregano and red-pepper chips. Include the chicken, zip the beat of the sack and grant it a speedy shake to combine. Fridge for at slightest 1 hour and up to 12 hours.
- Pre-heat a cast press to medium high warm. Evacuate the chicken from the marinade and flame broil each chicken thigh for 4-5 minutes on each side until done. Remove and set aside to rest.
- Cut the chicken against the grain into lean strips and exchange back into the skillet and sauté for 2 minutes until fair marginally fresh around the edges.
- Exchange the chicken to an expansive bowl and hurl to with the serving of mixed greens fixings and serve with the Lemon Oregano Vinaigrette

To create the cured ruddy onions

- Whisk to begin with 3 fixings and 1 glass water in a little bowl until sugar and salt break up. Put onion in a container; pour vinegar mix over.
- Let sit at room temperature for 1 hour some time recently utilizing. Moreover, can be made 2 weeks ahead. Cover and chill. Deplete onions some time recently utilizing.

NOTES

Make the onions at slightest an hour ahead so they pickle, but you'll be able moreover keep them for up to 2 weeks.

Flame broiled Chicken with Avocado Tomato Serving of mixed greens

Barbecued Chicken with Avocado Tomato Serving of mixed greens checks off all the boxes when it comes to a supper party feast! It's lovely, integral inviting, scrumptious and most critical Simple! This flame broiled chicken supper party feast is past. Marinated flame broiled chicken combined with a fantastic avocado tomato and corn serving of mixed greens is the foremost culminate summer chomp.

Fixings

For the Chicken:

- ¼ glass extra-virgin olive oil
- ¼ container new lime juice
- 1 tablespoon ground cumin
- ½ teaspoon legitimate salt
- ½ teaspoon crisply ground dark pepper
- 4 chicken breasts with skin

For the Topping:

- 2 avocados cut into wedges
- 3-4 legacies tomatoes cut into ½ inch cuts
- 2 corn on the cob
- 1 formula Cilantro Vinaigrette

Informational

- Combine the fixings for the chicken marinade in a bowl and mix to combine. Include the chicken and marinate for 30-45 minutes at room temperature.
- Warm a flame broil to tall warm. Lift chicken from marinade (dispose of marinade) and flame broil chicken, turning frequently, until not pink in center, 10 to 15 minutes.

- Exchange chicken to a platter and best with the avocados, cherry tomatoes and crude corn cut off the cob. Present with the cilantro vinaigrette and season with salt and pepper.

NOTES

Not a fan of cilantro? Attempt a basil vinaigrette instep.

Chicken Parmesan

The foremost idealize and straightforward recipe for Chicken Parmesan! The leading dinner for date evenings at domestic, a simple family supper or an Italian themed supper party!

Fixings
- 1 24-ounce bump of your favorite tomato based pasta sauce
- 4 boneless skinless chicken breast beat lean to approximately ½ inch
- ½ container all reason flour
- 3 eggs beaten with 2 tablespoons water and prepared with salt and pepper
- 1 glass Italian prepared panko breadcrumbs
- ¼ glass olive oil
- 1 lb new mozzarella daintily cut
- ½ glass crisply ground parmesan
- Kosher salt and naturally split dark pepper to taste
- Pasta or Serving of mixed greens on the side to serve

Informational
- Preheat broiler to 400 degrees F.
- Season chicken on the two sides with salt and pepper. Dig each breast in the flour and tap off any abundance flour, at that point

plunge within the egg blend and let overabundance trickle off, at that point dig on both sides within the bread pieces.
- Warm oil in a huge cast press dish and warm over tall warm until nearly smoking. Include 1 or 2 chicken breasts to the skillet, in any case many will fit and cook until brilliant brown on both sides, almost 2 minutes per side. Exchange to a plate and rehash with the remaining chicken breasts.
- Once the chicken is cooked, carefully wipe out the abundance oil and brown bits from the cast press skillet and include ½ of the pasta sauce within the foot of an expansive skillet. In the event that the skillet doesn't fit all the chicken breasts, utilize a huge heating dish instep.
- Include the skillet browned breaded breasts on beat of the pasta, and spoon the rest of the sauce over the chicken alongside a couple of cuts of the new mozzarella, salt and pepper, and break even with sums of the naturally ground parmesan. Transfer to the pre-heated broiler and heat until the chicken is cooked through and the cheese is liquefied, approximately 8-10 minutes. Evacuate from the stove and decorate with basil. Serve over a bowl of pasta.

NOTES

Usually continuously delicious with pasta, but you'll continuously skip the carbs and serve with a basic serving of mixed greens.

Chicken Parmesan Meatballs
Fixings & Substitutions
- Ground Chicken
- Parmesan ground

- Panko Breadcrumbs
- Egg
- Salt
- Black Pepper crisply split
- Dried Oregano
- Dried Parsley
- Ruddy Pepper Drops
- Flour
- Bocconcini Mozzarella Balls
- Olive Oil
- Basil Takes off

How to Form Chicken Parm Meatballs

Stage 1: In a sweeping mixing bowl, consolidate the chicken, parmesan, breadcrumbs, egg, salt, pepper, oregano, parsley and reddish pepper pieces. Carefully combine everything together with your hands until the fixings are equitably blended.

Step 2: Shape the ground chicken blend into little meatballs, each the size of a golf ball. Embed a little bocconcini ball within the center of each meatball, taking care to change the meatball around the cheese once it's been embedded. The mozzarella ought to be totally covered up from locate.

Step 3: Dredge each meatball within the flour to softly coat it and delicately tap off any abundance flour. Preheat the broiler to 350 degrees F.

Step 4: Warm the olive oil in an expansive overwhelming foot skillet over medium tall warm. When the oil is hot, incorporate portion of the meatballs and sauté for a 3-4 minutes, turning each so routinely to brown the outside.

Step 5: Once all meatballs are browned, include the tomato sauce to the skillet and put the browned meatballs on top of the sauce.

Stage 6: Move the skillet, meatballs and all, into the grill and let the meatballs continue to plan for 15-20 minutes until cooked through.

Evacuate the skillet from the stove and tidying with salt, pepper, freshly chopped basil and extra bocconcini in the event that craved. Serve quickly.

Chicken Parmesan Gnocchi Prepare
Fixings & Substitutions
- Plain Gnocchi
- Additional Virgin Olive Oil
- Yellow Onion
- Garlic
- Legitimate Salt
- Black Pepper crisply split
- Ground Chicken

How to Make Chicken Parmesan Gnocchi Heat

Step 1: Preheat the broiler to 425 degrees F. Heat a tremendous pot of water to the point of boiling. Include the gnocchi to the bubbling water and cook concurring to the bundle headings; deplete, saving ¼ cup of the cooking fluid.

Step 2: Meanwhile, heat the oil in a large nonstick cast press skillet over medium-high warm. Include the onions and garlic and cook, blending sometimes, until delicate, almost 5 minutes.

Step 3: Include the ground chicken and cook, mixing sometimes, until the chicken is cooked through and the onions are brilliant brown, 10 to 12 minutes. Remove from the warm and season with salt and pepper.

Step 4: Include the gnocchi, saved cooking fluid, marinara sauce and ruddy pepper chips to the skillet with the chicken blend and mix to combine.

Step 5: Add the parmesan and stir.

Step 6: Sprinkle with the mozzarella. Heat on the beat stove rack until hot and bubbling and the cheese turns brilliant, almost 15 minutes.

Step 7: Evacuate from the broiler and let sit for 5 minutes. Add the burrata on beat.

Furthermore, season with salt and pepper as required. Decorate with new herbs and serve.

Spaghetti Squash Chicken Parmesan Bake
Fixings
- 1 medium spaghetti squash, divided the long way and seeds evacuated
- 3 tablespoons olive oil, divided
- 1 medium yellow onion, diced
- 6 cloves garlic, roughly chopped
- kosher salt and naturally split dark pepper
- 1 pound ground chicken
- 2 glasses marinara sauce
- ½ teaspoon smashed ruddy pepper drops
- 1 container destroyed mozzarella
- ½ glass destroyed parmesan
- 1 ball burrata cheese
- fresh basil or oregano to decorate

Enlightening
- Preheat the grill to 475 degrees F.

- Place the prepped spaghetti squash on a preparing sheet, cut side up, and sprinkle with olive oil, salt and pepper and broil until fork delicate and effortlessly shreddable, almost 45-60 minutes. Expel and carefully shred the squash and transfer to a bowl Warm the oil in a huge nonstick cast press skillet over medium-high warm. Include the onions and garlic and cook, mixing sometimes, until delicate, almost 5 minutes. Add the ground chicken and cook, mixing incidentally, until the chicken is cooked through and the onions are splendid brown, 10 to 12 minutes. Empty from the warm and prepare with salt and pepper.
- Include the spaghetti squash, marinara sauce and ruddy pepper drops to the skillet with the chicken mixture and blend to combine. Include the parmesan and blend.
- Sprinkle with the mozzarella. Bake on the beat broiler rack until hot and bubbling and the cheese turns brilliant, almost 15 minutes. Expel from the stove and let sit for 5 minutes. Include burrata on best. What's more, season with salt and pepper as required. Embellish with fresh herbs and serve

NOTES

The spaghetti squash acts unequivocally like a pasta and ingests the kinds of the chicken parmesan mix greatly. Everything gets prepared into a skillet or casserole dish and topped with cheese. You'll indeed go so far as to serve it with burrata in the event that you need to be additional wanton!

Mushroom Chicken Parmesan Pasta
Fixings
- 1 lb spaghetti

- 2 tablespoons olive oil
- 1 pound crimini or infant bella mushrooms finely dice
- 2 cloves garlic finely chopped
- 1 pound ground chicken
- 1 teaspoon legitimate salt
- ¼ teaspoon dark pepper
- 1 14.5-ounce can diced tomatoes undrained
- 1-2 cups marinara sauce (I utilized a tomato basil pasta sauce from Rao's)
- ½ glass ground Parmesan
- ¼ container chopped chives

Informational

- Cook the pasta as indicated by the bundle bearings. Deplete and return the pasta to the pot.
- Meanwhile, warm the oil in a large pan over medium warm. Include the mushrooms and cook, mixing every so often, for 4-5 minutes until brilliant brown.
- Include the garlic, chicken, salt, and pepper and cook until the chicken is completely done.
- Spoon off and dispose of any fat. Incorporate the tomatoes and their juices and the tomato basil pasta sauce and heat to the point of boiling.
- Decrease warm and mix in half of the Parmesan. Stew until the sauce has thickened slightly, approximately 5 minutes. Include the sauce to the pasta and toss. Exchange to a large bowl or serve within the skillet.

NOTES

Utilize anything mushroom assortment looks great at the showcase.

Chicken Parmesan Pizza

This pizza is basically too great to share. It's heaped high with fresh mozzarella, juicy tomatoes, and breaded chicken and sprinkled with a bit of oregano and after that cleaned with salt and pepper.

INGREDIENTS
- 1 pound pizza mixture
- 2 eggs
- 1 container panko bread pieces
- 4 tablespoons shredded parmesan cheese
- 1 chicken breast beat into a ½ inch thickness
- 1 glass store bought pizza sauce
- 1 pound new mozzarella meagerly cut
- ½ container cherry tomatoes split
- 2 teaspoons dried oregano
- Fresh basil
- salt and pepper and ruddy pepper drops to taste

Informational
- Preheat your stove to 475 degrees F. Put the pizza batter on an oiled baking sheet and let rest for at slightest 30 minutes at room temperature.
- Whisk the eggs together in a medium measured bowl and set aside.
- Combine the panko breadcrumbs and destroyed parmesan cheese in another bowl and set aside.

- Plunge the piece of chicken into the egg mixture until it is fully coated. At that point plunge it in the bread piece blend and make beyond any doubt the bread scraps follow to the whole chicken breast. Put the chicken breast in a medium skillet over medium high warm with a couple of tablespoons of olive oil and cook for 4-5 minutes on each side until brilliant brown Expel the chicken and let rest on a paper towel to retain any abundance oil. Once cool, at that point cut into thin strips and set aside.
- In the meantime, roll the pizza dough out into 2 rounds. Evenly spread the pizza sauce on the batter and beat with cut chicken, cheese and tomatoes, at that point sprinkle with oregano and salt and pepper.
- Exchange the pizzas into the broiler and cook for 10-12 minutes until the cheese starts to bubble and turn brilliant brown. Evacuate the pizza from the broiler, decorate with basil at that point cut and serve.

Chicken Parmesan Panini

This Chicken Parmesan Panini may be a pack and go lunch everybody will cherish. What's way better than an impeccably cooked breaded chicken breast, with bubbly mozzarella on beat, slathered in tomato sauce and pesto, and squeezed between 2 pieces of ciabatta?

Fixings

For the Chicken Parmesan

- Marinara Sauce - utilize your favorite here

- Boneless Skinless Chicken Breasts - make beyond any doubt you pound at that point with a hammer until it's approximately ½ inch thick all through
- All-purpose Flour - the primary breading step, makes a difference the eggs follow to the chicken
- Eggs - beat them with 2 tablespoons water and season with salt and pepper
- Italian Prepared Panko Breadcrumbs - the key to super fresh chicken
- Vegetable Oil - for singing
- New Mozzarella - nothing is way better than GOOEY brilliant pools of mozzarella cheese.
- Crisply Ground Parmesan Cheese - wouldn't be chicken pram without it
- Legitimate salt and crisply split dark pepper - goes without saying
- For the Panini
- 4 little rolls ciabatta - or 8 cuts of your favorite dried up bread
- New Mozzarella - more cheese duh
- Basil Pesto - truly makes this Chicken Parmesan Panini sparkle
- Additional Marinara Sauce - utilize as needed
- How to form a Chicken Parmesan Panini
- Begin by preheating the stove to 400º F and warming the vegetable oil over medium tall warm in a large skillet. You need to form beyond any doubt the oil is hot some time recently including your chicken to the dish so it gets fresh.
- Whereas the oil warms up, put each chicken breast into an expansive plastic zip top bag, one at a time, and pound the chicken with a hammer until it's almost ½ inch thick all through. This step guarantees it cooks equitably, so do not skip it.

- Following, plan a breading station, one bowl of flour, one bowl of whisked eggs (include 2 tablespoons of water and season with salt and pepper) and one bowl of panko bread crumbs. Pat each chicken breast dry with a paper towel and after that plunge into the flour blend, taken after by the egg blend, and finally the bread pieces.
- Carefully put the chicken in hot oil over medium high heat and cook for around 2 minutes until the bread pieces are brilliant brown. Employing a match of tongs, flip the chicken over and let it proceed to cook on the inverse side. Once the chicken is fully cooked, expel it from the dish and set it on a paper towel lined plate to rest. Rehash this handle with the remaining chicken.
- Once all the chicken is cooked, carefully wipe out the overabundance oil and brown bits from the cast press skillet and include ½ of the pasta sauce within the foot of a huge skillet. On the off chance that the skillet doesn't fit all the chicken breasts, use a huge heating dish instep. Include the chicken on best of the sauce, and spoon the rest of the sauce over the chicken at the side a couple of cuts of the new mozzarella, salt and pepper, and break even with sums of the naturally ground parmesan. Transfer to the pre-heated stove and prepare until the chicken is cooked through and the cheese is softened, around 8-10 minutes. Expel from the broiler and set aside whereas you prep the Panini.
- Preheat your Panini press, and begin amassing the Panini's. Slice the ciabatta rolls in half. Oil or margarine the sides of the bread. On one piece of bread, include a little spoonful of pesto and on the other tomato sauce. Incorporate the chicken parm cutlet on the pureed tomatoes slice of bread and afterward add extra cheddar. Best with the other pesto slathered slice of bread and painstakingly put the panini in a warmed panini press. Near the panini press and cook for

4-5 minutes until the bread has flame broil marks and it's slight toasted. Rehash with the remaining Chicken Parmesan Paninis.

Varieties and Substitutions

- Vegetable Oil - Utilize anything oil you've got on hand, canola oil or any other oil with a tall smoke-point is best for singing.
- Bread Scraps - I love utilizing panko breadcrumbs but you'll too utilize Italian breadcrumbs.
- Fresh Mozzarella - In case you do not have new mozzarella you'll be able completely utilize ground mozzarella.
- Ciabatta - A dried up loaf of French bread would moreover work.

Corny Chicken and Rice Casserole

Fixings & Substitutions

- White Rice
- Annihilated Colby Jack & Mozzarella Cheese - At whatever point I require destroyed cheese I like to purchase it in a block and shred it myself. It's more fresh and softens way better in my supposition. I utilize Colby Jack and mozzarella in this Chicken and Rice Casserole formula since it dissolves so delightfully, but Monterey Jack or Pepper Jack would also work wonderfully!
- Refried Beans
- Solidified Charred Corn
- Yellow Onions
- Chopped Green Chiles
- Tomatillo Salsa
- Destroyed Rotisserie Chicken

- Salt & Pepper
- Scallions
- Cilantro

How to Form Tacky Chicken and Rice Casserole

Step 1: Preheat the stove to 375° F. Cook the rice agreeing to the bundle bearings. Once cooked, evacuate from warm and exchange the cooked rice into a huge bowl.

Step 2: Fold in 1 ½ cups of the destroyed colby jack cheese, ½ glass of the destroyed mozzarella, corn, onions, chicken, green chiles and salsa. Season the whole mixture with salt and pepper and blend to combine.

Step 3: Softly splash a medium measured skillet with non-stick shower, and line the foot with the refried beans. Transfer the blend into the skillet.

Step 4: Beat with the remaining destroyed cheeses and heat for almost 20-25 minutes until the top layer of cheese is bubbly and melted.

Step 5: Expel the heating dish from the broiler and garnish the Tacky Chicken and Rice Casserole with green onions and cilantro and serve.

Asian Chicken Slaw

Here is the arrangement with this Asian Chicken Slaw... It's impossible. Epic. So good you'll want to lick the foot of the bowl fair to form beyond any doubt that each last bit of goodness has been devoured and none is left to squander. And you can make it veggie lover fashion or with chicken.

Fixings & Substitutions

- Rice Wine Vinegar
- Soy Sauce
- Lime

- Shelled nut Butter
- Garlic
- Napa Cabbage
- Ruddy Cabbage
- Red Chime Pepper
- Yellow Chime Pepper
- Carrot
- Green Onions
- Avocado
- New Basil
- New Cilantro
- Destroyed Chicken Breast

How to Make Asian Chicken Slaw

Step 1: Whisk together the rice wine vinegar, soy sauce, lime juice, shelled nut butter and garlic until smooth.

Step 2: Combine the Napa cabbage, ruddy cabbage, cut chime peppers, carrot and green onion and hurl together.

Step 3: Include in a modest bunch of avocado, cut basil and new cilantro along with the destroyed chicken.

Step 4: Pour the fluid blend over the vegetables and chicken and hurl to combine. Season with additional soy sauce in the event that required and serve instantly.

Easy Chicken Pot Pie
Fixings & Substitutions

- Rotisserie Chicken – Using a rotisserie chicken in this formula could be a gigantic timesaver.
- Butter – All of the veggies get sautéed in butter, which makes this filling indeed more tasty. I like to utilize unsalted butter so you'll be able control how much salt you need to add to the formula.
- Vegetables – The classics include yellow onion, carrots, celery, solidified peas, and freshly minced garlic.
- Flour – All-purpose flour is included to the vegetables to form a roux which can offer assistance thicken the filling as it stews.
- Chicken Stock + Entirety Drain + Sherry – All three include indeed more flavor to the chicken pot pie filling and make a super smooth and gravy-like consistency.
- Herbs – Thyme, sage, chives, and parsley offer assistance brighten up the wanton filling.
- Panko Bread Scraps – Panko bread pieces are included to coat the foot of the dish some time recently pouring in the filling to act as the foot outside. You may do another layer of puff baked good, but to be genuine, typically less demanding and I incline toward it a bit lighter!
- Puff Baked good Sheet – Another awesome timesaver is utilizing store-bought solidified puff baked good sheets as the top crust. Puff baked good is super light, flaky, and works wonderfully as a pie outside. Fair be sure to let it defrost beneath refrigeration some time recently utilizing.

How to Make Chicken Pot Pie

Step 1: liquefy the butter over medium tall warm in an expansive Dutch Oven. Once softened, add the onion, celery and carrots. Sauté the vegetables for 5-7 minutes or until they gotten to be translucent. Include the garlic and cook for 60 seconds.

Stage 2: Diminish intensity to medium and sprinkle the flour over the veggies to make a roux. Cook out the flour for approximately 1-2 minutes until it begins to turn brilliant.

Step 3: Combine the chicken stock, drain and sherry in a little bowl. Once combined, gradually include the blend to the vegetables, blending to join. Let the blend come to a stew until it thickens, approximately 5 to 6 minutes.

Step 4: Once thickened, include within the shredded chicken, peas, and herbs and mix to combine. Taste and adjust salt and pepper on a case by case basis.

Step 5: Sprinkle the panko into the foot of a 9x13 dish to evenly coat the foot.

Stage 6: Pour the filling on top of the panko and let sit for 10 minutes to fairly cool.

Step 7: While the mixture is cooking, utilize a rolling pin to roll out the sheet of puff cake into an 11 x 15-inch rectangle, you need it fair somewhat bigger that the surface area of your preparing dish. In a little bowl, whisk together the egg yolk and water to make an egg wash.

Step 8: Carefully lay the sheet of puff pastry on beat of the heating dish and brush the surface of the baked good with the egg wash. Tuck any abundance mixture into the sides of the preparing dish to create an outside and pleat the edges. Sprinkle a couple of Malden salt on best of the puff cake/egg wash and after that painstakingly cut a little cuts in the surface to allow any examine to elude.

BBQ Chicken Quinoa Serving of mixed greens

This Stacked BBQ Chicken Quinoa Serving of mixed greens is one of my favorite make ahead dinners!!

Fixings

- 1 ½ glasses cooked quinoa
- ½ glass new corn cut from the cob
- ½ glass dark beans washed and depleted
- 1 glass destroyed BBQ chicken can utilize a store bought chicken and hurled with a small BBQ sauce
- 1 avocado chopped
- 3-4 tablespoons White Cheddar cheese destroyed
- BBQ sauce
- 2 scallions chopped
- cilantro for decorate

Enlightening

- In a huge bowl, hurl together the quinoa, corn, dark beans, chicken and avocado. Season with salt and pepper
- Exchange blend onto a bowl and beat with destroyed cheese, BBQ sauce, scallions and cilantro.
- Serve

NOTES

This formula calls for as of now cooked chicken so arrange ahead! In case I have time, I incline toward to cook my chicken within the crockpot, utilizing 6 chicken thighs, 1 white onion cut and ½ container of BBQ sauce. I cook on moo for about 6-7 hours and after that shred and refrigerate for afterward.

Barbecued BBQ Chicken Pizza

Your favorite flavors from BBQ Chicken onto a pizza with a barbecued pizza hull! You will be fixated.

Fixings

- 1 lb pizza mixture
- olive oil for brushing
- ½ container store bought BBQ sauce
- Fresh mozzarella cheese torn
- 1 glass destroyed cooked chicken
- ½ glass corn cut off the cob
- ¼ ruddy onion meagerly cut
- ½ container split cherry tomatoes
- small modest bunch of cilantro
- small modest bunch of chopped green onions
- legitimate salt and normally split dim pepper to taste

Enlightening

- Plan a gas or charcoal grill to tall warm. Brush the flame broil with a bit of oil.
- Shape the batter into 2 medium-ish pizzas whereas on a clean floured surface. Let the dough sit for 5 minutes and after that re-form to create beyond any doubt it's as huge as you'd like. Place the pizza batter on a delicately floured rimless preparing sheet, or pizza peel.
- Exchange the mixture over to the barbecue, and slide the pizza dough directly onto the flame broil. Barbecue the mixture for approximately 2 minutes with the cover closed. Utilizing a match of tongs, lift the cover, and flip the mixture over onto the other side and

cook for approximately 2 minutes more. The mixture ought to be brilliant brown with grill marks on both sides.
- Once the batter is cooked, expel it from the barbecue and put it back onto the preparing sheet.
- Brush the olive oil over the beat side pizza and after that spread the BBQ. Orchestrate the mozzarella, destroyed chicken, corn and ruddy onion and put back onto the barbecue until the cheese has softened.
- Utilizing tongs, expel the pizza from the barbecue and season with salt and pepper as required. Best with the cherry tomatoes, cilantro, green onions and serve quickly.

NOTES
As long as you let it "set up" your pizza outside shouldn't be stuck to the grates once you go to flip it.

Ginger Scallion Chicken Wraps
Some of the time you fair require a speedy and simple weeknight supper and these Ginger Scallion Chicken Wraps are precisely that!
Fixings
- ½ head napa cabbage destroyed
- ½ head purple cabbage destroyed
- 1 yellow chime pepper cut into matchsticks
- 1 ruddy chime pepper cut into matchsticks
- ½ english cucumber cut into matchsticks
- 6 ounces shitake mushrooms cut
- 2 tablespoons vegetable oil
- 2 cooked chicken breasts destroyed

For the Ginger/Scallion sauce:
- 1 bunch scallions daintily cut (around 1 ¼ glass add up to)
- 1 3- inch piece of ginger peeled and exceptionally finely minced
- 4 cloves garlic minced
- 4 teaspoons toasted sesame oil
- 8 tablespoons soy sauce
- 4 tablespoons rice vinegar
- ⅓ glass vegetable oil
- 1 teaspoon ruddy pepper chips

To Wrap
- 4 Expansive Spinach tortilla wraps

Informational
- In a huge bowl combine the napa cabbage, purple cabbage, yellow and ruddy chime pepper and cucumber.
- In a medium skillet, saute the mushrooms within the oil until brilliant brown. Once brilliant, expel and include to the cabbage blend along with the destroyed chicken breasts.
- Consolidate the elements for the Ginger Scallion sauce in a bowl. Put half of the sauce aside to utilize for plunging, and combine the remaining half with the cabbage blend and hurl to combine.
- Orchestrate the 4 huge spinach tortilla wraps on a clean surface. Spoon rise to sums of the cabbage chicken blend in the center of each wrap and wrap (like chipotle) to seal. Cut in half and serve quickly.

NOTES

Feel free to utilize more of the sturdy lettuce and skip the wraps.

Poblano Chicken Enchiladas

These have bounty of enchilada sauce and bountiful sums of cheese. Incorporate to that a delectable filling of obliterated chicken, poblano peppers and corn and it's a triumphant blend.

Fixings
- 2 teaspoons vegetable oil
- 1 ruddy onion cut
- 1 poblano or pasilla pepper cut
- 1 container corn
- 14 oz diced green chiles 1 can
- 2 cloves garlic generally chopped
- 1 teaspoon cumin
- ½ teaspoon chili powder
- 12 corn tortillas
- 1 rotisserie chicken shredded
- 2 cans 15 ounces Ruddy Enchilada Sauce
- 1 ½ container destroyed Monterey jack cheese
- 1 ½ container destroyed cheddar cheese

Garnishes:
- Sour Cream, Pico de gallo, Chopped Chives, New Cilantro

Enlightening
- Preheat the stove to 350 F.
- In a large skillet, warm the oil over medium tall warm. Include the onions and poblano peppers and saute for 5-6 minutes until delicate. Incorporate the corn, green stew peppers, garlic, cumin and bean stew powder and saute for various minutes more until the vegetables are caramelized. Include the chicken and blend to combine.

- Evacuate the vegetable blend from the skillet and set it aside. Pour the enchilada sauce into the same skillet and decrease the warm to moo, permitting it to warm through.
- Pour 1 cup of warmed sauce into the foot of a casserole dish.
- To accumulate the enchiladas, dive a tortilla into the sauce by then lay on a plate. Sprinkle a bit of each sort of cheese down the center, taken after by a few of the destroyed chicken/vegetable blend. Roll it up firmly, at that point put it, crease side down, within the dish. Rehash with the rest of the tortillas.
- Pour the rest of the sauce over the enchiladas, at that point sprinkle on the rest of the cheese. Exchange to the broiler and heat it for 30 minutes, or until hot and bubbly.
- Expel the dish from the oven and decorate with any garnishes as required. Serve immediately.

NOTES

You'll make them additional energetic by adding any number of fixings from pico de gallo, new cilantro, sour cream, chives, more cheese... you title it! It's basically all my favorite things rolled up into a culminate small tortilla circumstance!

Thai Chicken Pizza

This Thai Chicken Pizza has been on significant upheaval! All you wish is a few extra rotisserie chicken and a speedy shelled nut sauce and you're in commerce.

Fixings

For the Peanut Sauce

- 1 1-inch piece ginger peeled
- 1 little garlic clove
- ½ container velvety shelled nut butter
- 2 tablespoons soy sauce
- 1-2 tablespoons new lime juice
- 1 teaspoon stuffed light brown sugar
- ¼ -½ teaspoons pulverized ruddy pepper chips

For the Pizza
- 1 lb Pizza Dough
- 1 cup destroyed rotisserie Chicken
- 2 glasses Destroyed Mozzarella Cheese

For the Topping
- Green Onions
- Shredded Carrots
- Fresh Cilantro
- White Bean Sprouts
- Limes

Enlightening

For the Sauce
- Include all the fixings into a blender and ⅓ container water and mix, including more water by tablespoonfuls in the event that required to lean, until smooth.

For the pizza
- Preheat stove to 450 degrees F. Press the pizza mixture into the shape of a medium measured sheet skillet.
- Spread ½ cup the shelled nut sauce on beat, taken after by the destroyed cheese and the diced chicken.

- Exchange to the broiler and heat until the cheese is dissolved and bubbly, around 10-15 minutes. Expel from the oven and best with TONS of the green onions, destroyed carrots, cilantro, bean grows and salt and pepper as required serve. Crush bounty of lime juice on best.

NOTES

Make your claim mixture or snatch a ball of arranged batter from the store counter. It's all tasty!

Custom made Chicken Taquitos

Keep in mind those solidified Chicken Taquitos you'd purchase as a kid - well these are hand crafted and they are Unimaginable!! You will be obsessed

Fixings

- 12 little corn tortillas
- 1 ½ glasses destroyed rotisserie chicken
- 1 chipotle in adobo, chopped + 1 tablespoon adobo sauce
- ½ teaspoon ground coriander
- Fit salt and freshly broken dim pepper to taste
- 2 glasses vegetable oil
- 1 lime

Serve with

- Arbol Salsa
- Mexican Crema
- Lime Wedges
- Cilantro
- Cotija

- Sliced Radishes

Enlightening

- Put destroyed chicken, chipotle in adobo and sauce, coriander and 1 teaspoon of salt and ½ teaspoons freshly broken dark pepper in a bowl, hurl to combine.
- To collect the taquitos you need the tortillas to be adaptable, in case your tortillas are on the stiff side you'll be able cover them with a moist towel and microwave for 10-15 seconds. Working with each tortilla in turn put a stacking tablespoon of chicken on the lower third of the tortilla spreading it to almost every one of the edges, crossover the tortilla over the chicken and roll firmly, secure with a toothpick. Keep the rolled taquitos beneath a soggy towel whereas rolling to maintain a strategic distance from cracking.
- Heat the oil in a cast iron skillet over medium tall warm. When oil is hot carefully put ½ of the taquitos into the oil and broil till brilliant brown, turning to cook both sides. Do not swarm the container. Add up to time almost 3-4 minutes.
- Expel taquitos from oil and deplete on a paper towel lined plate and sprinkle with a bit of legitimate salt and squeeze of lime. Rehash searing for remaining taquitos. Present with Mexican crema, arbol salsa and different garnishes

NOTES

Corn tortillas are significant for a bona fide taquito so skip the flour tortillas this time.

Greek Chicken Stuffed Pitas
Fixings & Substitutions

For the Tzatziki
- Plain Non-fat Greek Yogurt
- English Cucumber
- Lemon
- Garlic
- New Dill
- Kosher Salt
- Dark Pepper
- For the Stuffed Pita
- Rotisserie Chicken
- Tzatziki Sauce
- Ruddy Onion
- Hass Avocado
- Whole Wheat Pitas
- Legitimate Salt
- Dark Pepper

How to Form Greek Chicken Stuffed Pitas

Step 1: Combine everything into an expansive bowl but the lemon juice.

Step 2: Include half of the lemon juice and taste. Include more lemon juice if craved and season with salt and pepper as required.

Step 3: Put the pita bread in a toaster, toaster oven or broiler and toast for a few minutes until fair slightly toasty. Expel and set aside.

Step 4: Combine the cooked chicken, tzatziki sauce and ruddy onion in an expansive bowl and toss to combine. Taste and season with salt and pepper as required.

Step 5: Separate the blend into 4 rise to parts and stuff each into a pita stash and best with avocado cuts.

Green Chicken Enchiladas

Fixings

- Rotisserie Chicken - hot tip shred the chicken in your blender to save time though making these Green Chicken Enchiladas
- Flavors - I like to utilize ground coriander, ruddy pepper drops, and legitimate salt to season the chicken blend
- Vegetable Oil - safflower oil or avocado oil too works for warming the tortillas
- Flour Tortillas - you'll utilize corn tortillas.
- Cheese - I utilize a blend of destroyed Monterey Jack cheese and cotija cheese
- Crema - we're whipping up a speedy crema to sprinkle on beat of our enchiladas utilizing crème fraîche and a sprinkle of drain
- Hand crafted Tomatillo Sauce - the recipe is underneath and super simple to create, everything lovely much gets tossed into a blender
- Ruddy Onion and Cilantro - to decorate on beat of the Green Chicken Enchiladas

Varieties and Substitutions

- Green Enchilada Sauce – Whereas the homemade green enchilada sauce in this formula with shake your world you'll be able completely take a store-bought easy route and utilize your favorite bumped green enchilada sauce instep.
- Cheese – I adore a Montery Jack and Cotija cheese minute since it dissolves so flawlessly. Cheddar, Colby Jack, Pepper Jack, a Mexican-blend or anything comparative would too work magnificently!

- Flour Tortillas - Customarily enchiladas are made with corn tortillas, but you'll see that this formula calls for flour tortillas. Typically fair my individual inclination, I discover flour tortillas simpler to roll and less likely to break compared to corn tortillas. That being said, feel free to utilize corn tortillas in this formula.

How to Create Green Chicken Enchiladas

Step 1: Preheat the broiler to 425 degrees F. Sprinkle the olive oil over onion, poblano, and tomatillos on a heating sheet and cook until vegetables are delicate and browned, 35–40 minutes. Let cool somewhat some time recently peeling the skin off the poblano.

Step 2: Exchange the blend and any juices to a blender. Incorporate serrano chiles, garlic, chicken stock, cilantro, and lime juice and purée until smooth.

Step 3: Exchange to a huge bowl, then season with salt and pepper as required.

Step 4: Include the chicken with the ground coriander, ruddy pepper drops, and ½ glass green sauce in a huge bowl and season with salt and pepper.

Step 5: Hurl to combine.

Step 6: Warm vegetable oil in a medium skillet over medium-high. Working one at a time, broil the tortilla, turning once, approximately 5 seconds per side. Exchange tortilla to paper towels to deplete. Rehash with remaining tortillas.

Step 7: Plunge both sides of each tortilla in green sauce fair to coat, at that point exchange to a preparing sheet.

Step 8: Spread 1 cup green sauce longwise down the center of a 13×9" preparing dish. Working one at a time, spoon ¼ container of the chicken blend into the center of the tortilla and overlap one side over the filling, at that point proceed to roll the enchilada up like a burrito. Put crease side down within the arranged heating dish as you go, fitting them all in.

Step 9: Best with the remaining green sauce and after that heap on the cheese.

Step 10: Prepare until sauce is bubbling and cheese is starting to brown, 20–25 minutes.

Stage 11: Though the enchiladas are planning, join the crème fraîche and channel and season with salt.

Step 12: Serve enchiladas topped with cheese, a sprinkle of crema, cut onion and cilantro.

Tex Mex Enchilada Queso

This tacky Tex Mex Enchilada Queso completely, without a question, will be the MVP of your amusement day parties. It's fundamentally everything you'd toss into a bunch of enchiladas….but in plunge shape.

Fixings
- glass destroyed rotisserie chicken
- 8 ounces cream cheddar at room temperature
- 1 container acrid cream
- 1 tablespoon ground chili powder
- 1 teaspoon ground cumin
- ½ teaspoon garlic powder
- ½ teaspoon legitimate salt
- 1 10-ounce can Green Enchilada Sauce
- 1 15-ounce can dull beans, washed and draineds
- 1 10-ounce can diced tomatoes in green chilies, depleted
- 1 container frozen corn thawed

- 1 container naturally ground sharp cheddar cheese partitioned
- Chopped new cilantro
- Chopped green onions
- Nursery of Eatin'® Tortilla Chips for serving

Informational

- Preheat the broiler to 400°F.
- Gently coat a profound 9-inch skillet cooking splash.
- In a large bowl on medium speed, beat together the cream cheese, acrid cream, chili powder, cumin, garlic powder, and salt until smooth and well combined. Diminish speed to moo at that point beat within the enchilada sauce until joined. Blend within the beans, tomatoes, corn, ½ glass cheddar cheese, and destroyed chicken.
- Exchange the blend to the arranged baking dish. Beat with remaining ½ glass cheddar cheese. Heat for 25-30 minutes, until the plunge is hot and the cheese is bubbly. Sprinkle with cilantro and green onions, and serve warm with Plant of Eatin'® Tortilla Chips.

Firm Chicken Thighs with Crushed Peas

These Fresh Chicken Thighs with Crushed Peas are the extreme spring time supper formula!

Fixings

For the Chicken

- 6 bone-in skin-on chicken thighs
- Kosher salt and naturally ground pepper to taste
- 1 teaspoon ground coriander
- ½ teaspoon ground cumin

- 1 tablespoon olive oil

For the Peas
- 1 10-ounce bundle solidified peas, totally defrosted
- 4 cloves garlic, finely chopped
- ⅓ container finely ground Pecorino Romano cheese, also more to wrap up
- ⅓ container olive oil
- 2 lemons, 1 juiced and 1 cut
- ¼ teaspoon ruddy pepper pieces
- kosher salt and crisply split dark pepper
- fresh dill and new mint clears out, discretionary

Informational
- Position a rack within the lower third of an oven and preheat to 400°F
- Season the chicken thighs on the two sides with salt, pepper, cumin and coriander. Warm the oil in a huge ovenproof skillet over medium-high warm. Include the chicken, skin side down, and cook until the fat has rendered and the skin is fresh and brilliant brown, almost 8 minutes.
- Flip the chicken to the other side and scramble the lemon cuts on beat. Exchange to the stove and cook until an instant-read thermometer embedded into the thickest portion of a thigh, absent from the bone, registers 170°F (77°C), 18 to 20 minutes.
- Whereas the chicken is broiling, make the crushed peas. Exchange the garlic to a medium bowl and include the pecorino, olive oil, lemon juice, ruddy pepper chips, salt, and bounty of dark pepper, and whisk to combine. Add the defrosted peas and blend to combine. Taste and alter salt and pepper as required. Use the rear of a fork

and just for the most part squash half of the peas so they are a little more thick and remove the other half whole. Expel the chicken from the broiler, include the peas into the ovenproof skillet, basically nesting the chicken thighs into the peas and coating the peas with the chicken renderings and beat with herbs and additional lemon, salt and pepper.

NOTES

This can be the culminate feast to keep within the back of your intellect since it employments wash room and cooler fixings that are so easy to come by.

Butter Chicken

This super flavorful Butter Chicken couldn't be simpler to make! It's particularly tasty served with a warm piece of naan!

Fixings

For the Marinade

- 2 pounds boneless skinless chicken thighs or bosoms cut into 1 inch pieces
- 1 glass Stonyfield Grassfed Greek Quarts
- 2 tablespoons lemon juice
- 1 ½ tablespoons ground turmeric
- 2 tablespoons garam masala
- 2 tablespoons ground cumin
- 1 teaspoon cayenne pepper

For the remaining portion of the formula:

- ½ container butter
- 1 onion, generally diced
- 4 cloves garlic, roughly chopped
- 2 tablespoons new ginger, ground
- 1 15-ounce can diced tomatoes
- ½ glass chicken stock
- 2 glasses overwhelming cream OR coconut drain
- 1 teaspoon tomato glue
- 2 teaspoons salt
- Lemon juice to taste
- Cilantro to decorate
- Naan bread to serve

Informational
- Combine the chicken, greek yogurt, lemon juice, and flavors in a bowl. Marinate for at slightest 1 hour, or overnight.
- In a large pan over medium warm, soften the butter. Mix in onion and cook gradually until the onion and cook until translucent. Incorporate the garlic and ginger and cook until fragrant, around 2-3 minutes more.
- Include the tomatoes to the skillet and cook for 5 minutes. Include the chicken and its marinade to the dish and cook for 5 minutes. Include the chicken stock and bring the blend to a bubble - at that point lower warm and stew for 30 minutes. Blend within the heavy cream, tomato glue and salt and proceed to stew until the chicken has cooked through, approximately 15 minutes, and the sauce is thick.

- Taste, alter flavoring as required, include lemon juice for a bit of corrosive. Embellish with cilantro takes off and serve nearby warmed naan.

NOTES

I solidify littler parcels of this all the time, once it's completely cooked. In arrange to warm it, I fair evacuate it from the cooler, let it come to temp in the fridge and at that point exchange the blend to a non-stick skillet and re-heat over medium warm. It's an extraordinary dish to solidify since it re-heats so pleasantly!

Cuban Mojo Chicken Thighs

Fixings & Substitutions

- Garlic Cloves
- Shallot
- Legitimate Salt
- Lime Get-up-and-go
- Ground Cumin
- Dried Oregano
- Naturally Ground Dark Pepper
- Orange Juice
- Crisply Squeezed Lime Juice
- Additional Virgin Olive Oil

How to Create Cuban Mojo Chicken Thighs

Step 1: In a high-powered blender, combine all the marinade fixings and mix until smooth. Empty ⅓ compartment of marinade into a little bowl and save it for the plunging sauce.

Stage 2: Throw the chicken with the leftover 2 teaspoons of authentic salt and add the excess marinade. Marinate within the fridge for at slightest an hour and up to a day.

Step 3: Exchange the saved sauce to a non-stick skillet and reduce over medium tall warm for 3-5 minutes until thickened. Sprinkle over the flame broiled chicken and serve.

Step 4: Get ready a flame broil for medium tall warm, and delicately oil the barbecue grates. Place the chicken on the grates. Let the chicken char for 30-60 seconds and after that promptly diminish the warm to medium moo. Flame broil the chicken for approximately 10-15 minutes (or until the internal temperature comes to at slightest 165°F for thighs and 150°F to 155°F for breasts), turning each 5-7 minutes.

Thai Chicken Coconut Curry

This super delightful Thai Chicken Coconut Curry is the culminate make at domestic formula that you just can serve over rice!

Fixings
- 2 tablespoons coconut oil
- 1 onion, little dice
- 1 ruddy debutante pepper, little dice
- 4 cloves garlic, generally chopped
- 2 tablespoons new ginger, ground
- 1 ½ pounds boneless skinless chicken thighs, cut into 1 inch pieces
- 2 tablespoons curry powder
- 1 15 ounce can diced tomatoes
- ½ container chicken stock

- 2 glasses full fat coconut drain
- 1 teaspoon tomato glue
- 2 teaspoons salt
- Lime juice to taste
- Green Onions to decorate
- Cilantro to embellish
- White Rice for serving

Informational

- Put an expansive skillet over medium tall warm with the coconut oil.
- Include the onion and ruddy pepper sauté until fragrant, approximately 5 minutes.
- Incorporate the garlic and ginger and sauté for 30 seconds more.
- Include the chicken and curry powder and sauté until the chicken begins to turn brilliant brown, almost 10 minutes.
- Include the diced tomatoes, chicken stock, coconut drain, tomato glue and salt and bring to a bubble and decrease to a stew to proceed cooking until the chicken is completely cooked and the fluid thickens up.
- Taste, adjust flavoring as required, include lime juice to season and serve over rice with cilantro and green onions and additional lime wedges.

Chipotle Chicken Lettuce Wraps

These somewhat hot / smoky Chipotle Chicken Lettuce Wraps are rise to parts addictive and tasty!!

Fixings
- For the Chicken + Marinade
- 2 tablespoons olive oil
- 2 tablespoons water
- 3-4 chipotle peppers in adobo
- 1 teaspoon garlic powder
- 1 teaspoon ground cumin
- ½ teaspoon dried oregano
- ½ teaspoon dark pepper
- 10 boneless skinless chicken thighs cut down the middle

For the Lettuce Wraps:
- 1 head butter lettuce
- 2 mangos, cut into lean strips
- ½ ruddy onion, daintily cut
- ½ orange chime pepper, daintily cut
- 2 avocados, meagerly cut
- fresh mint
- fresh cilantro
- 1-2 limes, juiced
- Fit salt and freshly broken dull pepper to taste

Enlightening
- Put the ingredients for the marinade in a food processor or blender and mix until smooth. Coat the chicken thighs within the marinade and refrigerate for 1-4 hours.
- After marinating, Warm an indoor or open air barbecue to almost 400 degrees F (medium tall warm). Put the chicken onto the flame broil and barbecue 5 to 6 minutes per side, until the chicken is

cooked. Expel the chicken from the flame broil and let rest for 10 minutes.
- In the meantime - clean the butter lettuce and isolated it into glasses.
- Combine the mango, ruddy onion, chime pepper, avocado, mint, cilantro and lime juice in a bowl and hurl to combine. Season with salt and pepper.
- Collect the lettuce mugs with a bit of chicken, a few tablespoons of the topping and serve with additional limes in the event that required.

NOTES

Boston Bibb, green leaf, or romaine are my number one for lettuce wraps.

Chicken Shish Kabobs
Fixings
For the chicken:
- 3 tablespoons Gaby's Go To Flavoring
- 3 tablespoons extra-virgin olive oil
- 2 tablespoons ruddy wine vinegar
- 1 teaspoon coarse legitimate salt
- 1 teaspoon crisply ground dark pepper
- 6 garlic cloves roughly chopped
- 1 lemon juiced
- 1 lemon cut into wedges/sliced for serving
- 3 pounds boneless skinless chicken thighs and/or breasts cut into 1 ¼-inch 3d shapes
- 1 formula Basil Vinaigrette

Enlightening
- Combine the flavoring, olive oil ruddy wine vinegar, salt, pepper, garlic and lemon juice in a bowl; whisk to combine. Add in the chicken. Cover and chill at slightest 1 hour.
- Get ready barbecue over medium-high warm. String chicken pieces on sticks, isolating similarly. Dispose of marinade in bowl. Sprinkle each stick with extra Gaby's go-to flavoring.
- Barbecue chicken until brilliant brown and cooked through, turning sticks once in a while, 10 to 12 minutes add up to. Exchange sticks to platter. Present with basil vinaigrette and additional lemon wedge

Flame broiled Korean Chicken Sticks
Fixings
- ½ glass light brown sugar
- ½ glass unseasoned rice vinegar
- ¼ glass sambal oelek
- ¼ container soy sauce
- ¼ cup Sriracha
- 2 tablespoons finely grated peeled ginger
- 2 tablespoons finely chopped garlic
- 2 pounds skinless boneless chicken thighs, cut into 1 ½ inch pieces
- Sliced scallions for decorate
- Lime wedges for decorate

Informational
- Turn the Weber barbecue to medium-high warm.

- Whisk brown sugar, vinegar, sambal, soy sauce, Sriracha, ginger and garlic in an expansive bowl. Once combined, isolate similarly into two bowls. Include chicken to one of the bowls and hurl to coat. Let marinate for at slightest 30 minutes. Expel chicken and string 4 or 5 pieces onto each stick.
- Exchange the other bowl of the marinade (without the chicken) to a little pot. Bring to a bubble, decrease warm, and simmer until reduced by half, generally 7–10 minutes.
- Exchange the chicken to the flame broil, turning and seasoning regularly with diminished marinade, until cooked through, 8–10 minutes. Evacuate sticks and exchange to a serving platter. Sprinkle with the scallions and present with lime wedges.

NOTES

These would be glorify presented with rice and fire seared veggies.

Lemon Chicken Pasta

Meet the simple chicken pasta of your dreams! This Lemon Chicken Pasta is fair what you would like when you need to put supper on the table Quick!

INGREDIENTS
- 10 ounces linguini
- 2 tablespoons olive oil
- 5 cloves garlic generally chopped
- 1 shallot generally chopped
- 4 ounces shitake mushrooms cut
- 6 ounces crimini mushrooms cut
- 1 lb chicken thighs cut into 1 inch pieces
- 1 teaspoon ruddy pepper drops
- 1 bunch chives clipped

- 1 lemon zested and juiced
- handful of destroyed italian blend cheese
- kosher salt and crisply split dark pepper

Informational
- Bring a huge pot of water to a bubble. Cook pasta concurring to the bundle bearings, deplete and set aside.
- In a huge skillet, include the olive oil over medium high heat. Add the garlic, shallots and mushrooms and sauté for 6-7 minutes until delicate. Include the chicken and sauté until completely cooked - almost 10 minutes more. Season with salt, pepper and ruddy pepper drops.
- Once chicken is completely cooked, include the depleted pasta, lemon pizzazz, lemon juice and chives. Hurl everything together and alter flavoring as required. Serve with cheese blended in.

NOTES

Blend and coordinate your mushrooms with anything assortment looks the best at the advertise.

Shredded BBQ Chicken Burgers

The most straightforward Destroyed BBQ Chicken Burgers that you can make within the moderate cooker!!

Fixings
- 1 medium onion finely cut
- ½ glass ketchup
- ⅓ container cider vinegar
- ¼ container stuffed brown sugar

- ¼ glass tomato paste
- 2 tablespoons sweet paprika
- 2 tablespoons Worcestershire sauce
- 3 teaspoons legitimate salt
- 1 ¼ teaspoon crisply broken dark pepper
- 8-10 boneless skinless chicken thighs
- 6 ground sirloin sandwich buns
- 1 formula Guacamole
- 1 container destroyed colby jack cheese

Enlightening

- In your moderate cooker, combine the onion, ketchup, apple cider vinegar, brown sugar, tomato glue, paprika, Worcestershire, salt and pepper. Whisk to combine.
- Include the chicken thighs and make beyond any doubt they are all equitably spread out and coated with the sauce ingredients.
- Put the top on the moderate cooker and go to tall warm for the Annihilated bar-b-que Chicken to be exhausted 4-5 hours, and moo for Destroyed bar-b-que Chicken to be drained 7-8 hours.
- Once the clock is up, evacuate the lid and using 2 forks, shred the chicken while still in the container pot. Turn the container pot to warm and serve the Shredded BBQ Chicken on beat of burger buns with a piling spoonful of guacamole and shredded colby jack cheese.

NOTES

Then again - you may do this within the instant pot! Same bearings but tall weight for 20 minutes. Take off it alone for 10 minutes and after that discharge weight and shred with forks as required.

Hand crafted Orange Chicken

This hand crafted Orange Chicken is genuinely flawlessness!! So for those of you who arrange this each time you get takeout - attempt and make it and domestic and see what you think!

Fixings

For the Chicken

- 3 tablespoons cornstarch
- 3 egg whites
- 2 ½ lbs boneless skinless chicken thighs, cut into bite-sized pieces and tapped completely dry

For the Sauce

- ½ glass Orange Juice
- 1 tablespoon soy sauce
- 1 tablespoon brown sugar
- 1 tablespoon rice wine vinegar
- ¼ teaspoon sesame oil
- Kosher salt and pulverized ruddy pepper pieces
- 2 cloves garlic, finely chopped
- 1 teaspoon cornstarch
- vegetable oil for broiling
- green onion for decorate (or chives!)

INSTRUCTIONS

For the Chicken

- In a large bowl, whisk together the cornstarch and egg whites with a fork until almost foamy, about 1 miniature. Include the tapped dry chicken to the blend and permit to sit for 5 to 10 minutes.

For the Sauce

- Meanwhile, put the Squeezed orange, soy sauce, sugar, vinegar, sesame oil, salt, squashed red pepper and garlic in a little nonstick skillet and whisk. Warm until bubbling and beginning to thicken, approximately 5 minutes.
- Whisk together the cornstarch and ¼ glass water in a little bowl and include 1 to 2 tablespoons of the cornstarch slurry to the sauce. Blend in and thicken for 1 diminutive.
- Warm approximately 2-3 inches of vegetable oil in a large heavy-bottomed Dutch broiler until a deep-fry thermometer embedded within the oil registers 350 degrees F. In batches, carefully drop the chicken into the oil (I drop 1-2 pieces in at a time and move it around for a moment some time recently including more pieces), flipping delicately, until brilliant, 3 to 4 minutes. Be exceptionally cautious not to pack the skillet. Allow the pieces to exhaust on a plate fixed with paper towels for 2 to 3 minutes.
- Repeat the method with the remaining bunches. Once all the batches have their initial sear, drop them back into the oil for 1 diminutive to really set the coating. Hurl the chicken within the sauce and serve with the green onion embellish

NOTES

The chicken is not difficult to prepare and no you can't skirt the cornstarch. It's a crucial component in making it firm!! Too you wish to create beyond any doubt the chicken is smudged Completely dry some time recently including into the cornstarch egg white blend something else the coating wont adhere. This can be pivotal, particularly in case the chicken was already solidified and defrosted.

Artichoke Pepper Braised Chicken

Faultlessly moist chicken thighs braised in an artichoke and pepper sauce that is come full circle over rice, pasta or a bed of greens.

Fixings

- 4 tablespoons olive oil
- 6 bone-in chicken thighs
- Kosher salt and naturally broken dark pepper to taste
- 2 teaspoons ruddy pepper chips
- 1 huge yellow onion, peeled, divided and meagerly cut
- 6 cloves garlic, peeled and divided the long way
- 1 26-ounce jostle Gaby's Artichoke Pepper Sauce (or another artichoke pepper sauce of your choosing)
- cooked egg noodles hurled in butter to serve

Enlightening

- Warm the olive oil in a huge skillet or braiser over tall warm. Orchestrate the chicken thighs on a heating sheet and season them with salt and pepper, to taste. Turn the pieces on their other side and season once more. When the oil starts to smoke softly, carefully include the chicken, 3-4 pieces at a time to the oil. Permit them to brown on their to begin with side, almost 3 to 5 minutes. Utilize metal tongs to turn the chicken pieces to burn their moment side, almost 3 to 5 minutes. Trade the chicken to a spotless plate and put it away. Rehash with remaining chicken.
- Within the same skillet, add the chili chips, onions and garlic and mix to combine. Season the fixings with salt, to taste, at that point include the Artichoke Pepper Sauce. Stir to combine, and after that include the chicken back to the container, keep the warm moo and proceed cooking until the chicken is cooked through, 20 to 30 minutes. (If the sauce gets to be excessively thick or starts to stay to

the foot of the skillet, feel free to include a few water, almost ½ container at a time.)
- When the chicken is cooked through, evacuate from the warm and taste for flavoring. Serve nearby the cooked pasta or rice.

Fresh Lemon Chicken Thighs

A fast and easy dinner you'll be able count on! These chicken thighs are bound with bounty of citrus and new herbs – you'll be able wagered ever single chomp of these is reaching to be pressed with a pop of new flavor!

INGREDIENTS
- 6 bone-in, skin-on chicken thighs
- Genuine salt and freshly ground pepper to taste
- Fresh thyme
- Fresh tarragon
- 1 tablespoon vegetable oil
- ½ lemon cut into 8 rounds

Informational
- Position a rack within the lower third of an stove and preheat to 400°F
- Season the chicken thighs on the two sides with salt and pepper. Tuck many clears out of tarragon and thyme beneath the chicken skin. Warm the oil in an expansive ovenproof skillet or sear pan over medium-high warm. Include the chicken, skin side down, and cook until the fat has rendered and the skin is fresh and brilliant brown, about 8 minutes. Exchange, skin side up, to a plate.

- Pour off the overabundance fat from the dish. Return the chicken, skin side up, to the dish and scramble the lemon cuts on top. Transfer to the stove and cook until an instant-read thermometer embedded into the thickest portion of a thigh, absent from the bone, registers 170°F (77°C), 18 to 20 minutes.
- Exchange the chicken and lemon slices to a platter and scramble an extra 2-3 tablespoons of new herbs on beat. Let rest for 5 minutes some time recently serving.

NOTES

Bone-in chicken takes a shockingly long time to cook, so contribute in a great thermometer to guarantee your meat is cooked through.

Mushroom Chicken Marsala Pasta

One of those simple weeknight recipes that you'll need to form over and over once more!

Fixings
- 6 chicken thighs cut into nibble sized pieces
- 1 tablespoon olive oil
- 1 tablespoon butter
- Kosher salt and naturally broken dark pepper
- ½ teaspoon dried oregano
- 2 tablespoons all reason flour
- 1 container cut wild mushrooms
- 1 shallot generally chopped
- ½ container Marsala Wine

- ½ container Chicken Stock
- Fresh oregano for flavoring
- ½ lb fettuccine cooked

INSTRUCTIONS
- Warm the olive oil and butter in a sauté skillet.
- Season the chicken with salt, pepper, dried oregano and daintily dust with flour. Cook the chicken within the olive oil butter mixture for 8-10 minutes, mixing as often as possible until completely cooked. Expel to a plate and set aside.
- Include the chopped shallots and mushrooms to the skillet and sauté for 4-5 minutes until the mushrooms are brilliant brown. Deglaze with the Marsala and include chicken stock. Diminish the fluid until marginally thickened, almost 5 minutes. Return the chicken back into the dish and the cooked pasta and serve quickly. Diffuse the beat with new oregano.

NOTES

You'll utilize chicken breasts – but the chicken thighs are way more flavorful, pinkie guarantee! And the mushrooms may well be discretionary. You'll cherish each final nibble of this – I guarantee!

Brown Butter Chicken Pasta

Fixings
- 6 tablespoons Land O Lakes® Unsalted Butter isolated
- 2 pounds boneless skinless chicken thighs cut into pieces
- Kosher salt and crisply split dark pepper
- 2 tablespoons all-purpose flour

- 2 shallots thinly sliced
- 3 mugs cut mushrooms
- 8 garlic cloves minced or pressed
- ¾ glass dry white wine or chicken stock
- ½ pound long pasta
- ⅔ container naturally ground parmesan cheese + more for topping
- freshly chopped parsley or scallions for topping

Informational
- Heat a small pot over medium warm and include 3 tablespoons of butter. Whisk continually until butter has brown bits on the foot, at that point promptly expel from warm. Set aside.
- Warm a huge skillet on medium-high warm and include 1 tablespoon of butter. Pat chicken dry with a paper towel at that point hurl with salt, pepper and flour. Include the chicken to the skillet and brown on all sides, cooking for around 10-12 minutes total. Expel and set aside in a bowl. Turn heat down to moo and include the final 2 tablespoons butter. Add the cut mushrooms and shallots with a squeeze of salt whereas mixing once in a while. Cook until mollified – almost 15 minutes.
- Cook the pasta concurring to the bundle headings.
- Once the mushrooms and shallots are caramelized, include garlic and cook for 30 seconds until fragrant. Increase the warm to medium and include wine. Allow the wine to air pocket and cook for 2-3 minutes. Include chicken and pasta both to the skillet, hurling numerous times to coat. Turn off warm and blend in ground cheese. Sprinkle earthy colored spread (ensure you get the earthy colored bits!) up and over, throwing to cover several additional times. Serve with extra cheese and chopped parsley.

Chicken Paprikash

Chicken Paprikash could be a traditional Hungarian recipe and some way or another it can advance into the hearts of your loved ones. It's essentially stewed chicken in a paprika roux with tons of additional flavor from onions and garlic and herbs. Def a swarm pleaser no matter who you are serving it to!

Fixings

- 2 pounds boneless skinless chicken thighs (around 6-8 pieces), cut into little 1 inch pieces
- Kosher salt and naturally ground black pepper
- 2 tablespoons flour
- 1 huge yellow onion finely chopped
- 6 garlic cloves roughly chopped
- 3 tablespoons unsalted butter partitioned
- 3 tablespoons paprika
- ¼ teaspoon cayenne pepper
- 1 15- ounce can pulverized tomatoes
- ½ cup sour cream at room temperature
- 12 ounces egg noodles
- ½ glass parsley generally chopped

Informational

- Put chicken thighs on a plate and pat dry with paper towels. Season the chicken with salt and pepper and flour.
- Warm an expansive cast press skillet over medium-high. Include 1 tablespoon of butter. Using tongs, add chicken in and cook, hurl sometimes until completely cooked. Transfer chicken to a plate.

- Decrease the warm to moo and include the onion and garlic and season with salt and pepper. Cook, mixing frequently to break down browned bits on foot of skillet, until onions are translucent, 6–8 minutes.
- Include paprika and cayenne. Cook, blending continually, fair until onions are equitably coated and spices are fragrant, around 30 seconds. Include tomatoes to skillet. Fill can two-thirds with water and twirl, at that point include to skillet. Blend until joined, flavoring with salt as you blend, and bring to a simmer. Stew for 10 minutes. Using utensils, set up the chicken with any amassed juices back into the skillet and stew.
- Cook the egg noodles concuring to bundle informational, blending every so often. Deplete noodles and exchange to a huge bowl. Include the remaining 2 tablespoons of butter, and hurl to coat until butter is liquefied and noodles are coated. Season with salt and pepper.
- Finely chop ½ cup parsley and add half to noodles; hurl to coat.
- Taste sauce and season with salt and pepper depending on the situation. Spoon in a spoonful of the acrid cream and blend to combine. Proceed including the acrid cream, small by small so it doesn't sour. Include the cooked pasta into the mixture and include the remaining parsley on best.

NOTES

Make beyond any doubt you blend your acrid cream in bit by bit after the sauce is warmed. Doing this will offer assistance it remain smooth, consolidate easily, and not turn sour.

Chicken Tagine with Olives

The foremost delish Chicken Tagine with Olives adjusted from one of our visit guides in Morocco!

Fixings

For the Chicken

- 8 cloves garlic finely chopped
- 1 teaspoon sweet paprika
- 1 teaspoon ground cumin
- ½ teaspoon ground ginger
- ½ teaspoon saffron strings pulverized
- ½ teaspoon turmeric
- Genuine salt and normally ground dull pepper
- 6-8 bone in skin on chicken thighs

For the Tagine

- 2 tablespoons olive oil
- 3 yellow onions, daintily cut
- ¼ teaspoon ground cinnamon
- 16 green castelvetrano olives, set and crushed
- 1 lemon, peeled into thick cuts (employing a vegetable peeler to peel the lemon peel into thick 1 inch strips)
- 1 container chicken stock
- Juice of ½ lemon
- 1 tablespoon chopped flat-leaf parsley

Informational

- Mix garlic, saffron, ginger, paprika, cumin and turmeric alongside ½ teaspoon of salt and ½ teaspoon naturally broken dark pepper. Rub the chicken with blend, cover, and refrigerate to marinate for 3 to 4 hours.

- Warm oil in overwhelming skillet. Include chicken, and brown on all sides. Expel to plate and set aside. Include onions to skillet, and cook over medium-low heat almost 15 minutes, until they start to caramelize. Include the ground cinnamon and blend to combine.
- Put chicken on onions. Scramble with olives and the lemon strips. Scramble over chicken. Blend stock and lemon juice. Pour over chicken.
- Cover the skillet and put over moo warm, and cook around 30 minutes, until chicken is cooked through. Diffuse parsley on beat, and serve.

NOTES

Usually traditionally served on its claim, but you'll continuously include rice or bread on the off chance that you'd like something to drench up every last delightful drop.

Simple Mexican Destroyed Chicken {Verde!}

Culminate delicate, drop separated chicken simply can take and utilize for any number of things. Tacos – yes. Enchiladas – Duh. Burritos – completely. Taco Serving of mixed greens – why not. Quinoa Bowls – Clearly. The thoughts fair keep coming.

Fixings
- 6 boneless skinless chicken thighs
- Kosher salt and pepper
- 2 tablespoons olive oil
- 1 container Green Enchilada Sauce or Tomatillo Salsa

Enlightening
- Season the chicken thighs with salt and pepper on the two sides.

- Put a huge skillet with olive oil over tall warm and let the oil heat for a minute. Employing a match of tongs, include the chicken to the skillet and burn the chicken on both sides for 3 minutes each so that each side is brilliant brown.
- Include the Gentle Green Chile Enchilada Sauce to the skillet and cover the skillet with a tight fitting top. Diminish the warm to medium and let the chicken cook for 25-30 minutes.
- Following 20 minutes, using a match of utensils, flip the chicken over to the over side and continue to cook for an additional 10 minutes. Turn the warm off and utilizing 2 forks, shred the chicken and after that utilize as required.

For an Moment Pot
- Season the chicken thighs with salt and pepper on the two sides.
- Turn an moment pot onto the saute setting. Include the olive oil and let the oil warm for a minute. Utilizing a combine of tongs, include the chicken to the moment pot and burn the chicken on both sides for 3 minutes each so that each side is brilliant brown. Include the sauce or salsa on beat, near the top and make beyond any doubt it's fixed, and set the moment pot to poultry. Let the chicken cook and evacuate once the instant pot is done. Shred with 2 forks and serve as required.

NOTES

Utilize this chicken in tacos, enchiladas, or on burrito bowls.

Italian Wedding Soup
Fixings
For the Meatballs

- ½ pound ground chicken
- ¼ container ground parmesan
- ¼ container Italian breadcrumbs
- 1 egg
- ½ teaspoon legitimate salt
- ½ teaspoon crisply split black pepper
- ¼ teaspoon dried oregano
- ¼ teaspoon dried parsley
- ¼ teaspoon ruddy pepper chips
- 2 tablespoons olive oil

For the Soup
- 1 tablespoon olive oil
- 1 small onion, finely diced
- 4 cloves garlic, finely minced
- ¼ teaspoon ruddy pepper chips
- 8 glasses chicken or vegetable stock (moo sodium favored)
- 1 teaspoon legitimate salt
- ¼ teaspoon crisply broken dark pepper
- ½ bunch wavy kale, stems disposed of and greens torn into nibble estimate pieces, almost 4 mugs
- 1 egg
- 2 tablespoons ground parmesan, furthermore additional parmesan for serving
- 1 container cannellini beans, depleted and flushed
- 1 lemon, juiced

Informational

For the Meatballs

- In a broad mixing bowl, consolidate the chicken, parmesan, breadcrumbs, eggs, salt, pepper, oregano, parsley and pounded rosy pepper. Carefully combine everything along with your hands until the fixings are equitably blended.
- Shape the blend into little meatballs approximately 1 inch, almost 1 ½ teaspoon. Put on a preparing sheet.
- Warm the olive oil in an expansive skillet over medium tall warm and working in bunches in case required sear the meatballs on all sides until brilliant, about 5 min. Evacuate to a paper towel lined plate to deplete.

To Create the Soup
- In a 5-6 quart Dutch oven or pot heat the olive oil over medium tall warm and sauté the onions, garlic and ruddy pepper drops for 3-5 mins until delicate. Include broth, salt and pepper and bring to a stew. Decrease the warm to medium low, add kale to the pot and cook until the kale is wilted around 3 minutes.
- Include the meatballs to the pot together with the beans and stew 8 mins.
- In a little bowl whisk the egg and ground parmesan, gradually pour the egg blend into the soup whereas mixing.
- Include lemon juice and alter flavoring with more salt, pepper, or pulverized ruddy pepper.
- Serve with extra parmesan and a press of lemon juice.

Simple White Chicken Chili
Fixings & Substitutions

The regular suspects:
- olive oil, yellow onion and garlic - these are the base of beautiful much each formula
- I utilize chicken broth or stock to create the soup, but you can do it with vegetable stock on the off chance that that's what you have on hand.
- Diced green chilies - the tucson young lady in me will break out the green chilies on every occasion conceivable

Seasonings - a key portion of this formula and incorporate:
- ground cumin, ground coriander, dried oregano, stew powder, paprik and cayenne pepper. Nothing out of the conventional.
- New lime juice is key in this formula to really brighten things up once it's prepared to eat.
- Canned white beans - this includes a few bulk to the dish!
- Acrid cream is what I utilize to form this soup velvety. A parcel of times I've seen it with cream cheese which (whereas delish) isn't my stick for a soup!
- We need some corn (solidified or fresh) works!
- And final but not slightest, cooked shredded chicken. Buy a rotisserie from the store!!

How to Form White Chicken Chili

Step 1: Warm olive oil in an expansive overwhelming foot Dutch broiler over medium-high warm. Incorporate the onion and sauté until clear, just about 5 minutes.

Step 2: Include garlic and cook for 30 seconds.

Stage 3: Incorporate the flavors and saute until fragrant, 30 extra seconds.

Stage 4: Incorporate chicken stock, green chilies, lime squeeze and season with salt and pepper to taste. Include the ½ of the beans and blend to combine.

Utilizing your submersion blender, mix the blend for 10-20 seconds to puree. Same procedure as the Tortilla Soup on WGC!! Usually what makes it velvety.

Step 5: Include the remaining whole beans and corn to the dutch broiler. Bring the blend to a simmer and cook, revealed, for 15 to 30 minutes.

Step 6: Expel from warm and blend in acrid cream and cooked chicken.

Step 7: Serve embellished with cilantro, destroyed cheese, avocado slices and tortilla chips if desired.

Chicken Tortilla Soup
Ingredients/Substitutions

- Olive Oil- You can completely sub this fixing with another oil of your choice such as avocado oil, canola oil, etc.
- Onion- Onions include an additional kick of flavor to any formula and this one is no special case!
- Garlic- We cannot live without garlic. Drench in that captivating scent amid the primary few steps of this formula!
- Jalapeño- Cut jalapeños in the event that you want a bit of a kick
- Legitimate Salt and Dark Pepper- These two are a must in any recipe, they are so basic however so important!
- Dried Oregano- This flavor complements the rest of the flavors flawlessly!
- Cumin- Any sort of Mexican dish isn't total without this flavor! This is one of the key fixings to pull all the flavors together.

- Chipotle Pepper- We're including some spice to this formula since why not!? On the off chance that you'd rather keep the spice level mellow, you'll be able skip this zest.
- Fire Simmered Tomatoes and Green Chiles- These include SO much flavor to this formula. It gives a fair smokey flavor without a lot of flavor.
- Chicken Stock- If you need to skip the chicken totally and make this vegan - fair use vegetable stock and you're in trade.
- Dark Beans- While black beans are conventional in a Chicken Tortilla Soup, you may utilize Pinto Beans in case you incline toward!
- Solidified Corn- I like utilizing solidified corn for comfort but in the event that you favor to utilize canned or fresh corn, go for it!
- Rotisserie Chicken- Any sort of destroyed poultry works in this. Chicken is my favorite but on the off chance that you're making this and have extra turkey - be my visitor!!
- Cheese- Naturally destroyed cheese - I always opt for crisply shredded over the pre-shredded. It softens way better and it's fair more flavorful as it's naturally ground.
- Cilantro & Green Onion- New herbs like Cilantro, scallions or chives include a pleasant punch of flavor.
- Corn Tortillas-Firm tortilla strips or broke down up tortilla chips are the secret fixing with regards to chicken tortilla soup. The crunch really levels up the dish cherish making my possess chips and strips - utilize this as a direct.
- Limes- Lime juice - includes a small additional oomph
- Avocado- The avocado chunks includes a pleasant velvety touch to this soup without being overwhelming!

How to create this Chicken Tortilla Soup

Step 1: Turn on the stove to medium-high warm. Put an expansive pot on the stove and include the onion, garlic and jalapeño.

Step 2: Cook until the onion is see-through and the jalapeño is delicate. At that point include salt, pepper, dried oregano, cumin and chipotle pepper. Stir until it is all blended together and cook for 1-2 minutes more.

Step 3: Include fire broiled tomatoes and chicken stock to the container and hold up until it bubbles. At that point turn down the heat so it is just stewing and let it stew for 30 minutes without blending.

Stage 4: Following 30 minutes, use a submersion blender to make the soup smooth some time as of late including dim beans, corn and obliterated chicken into the pot.

Step 5 (discretionary): In a little skillet, heat the vegetable oil over medium tall warm. Once hot, add the tortilla strips in a single layer, singing rapidly for almost 30-45 seconds, flipping them once to guarantee both sides get fresh. Evacuate the tortillas once fresh with a match of tongs and transfer them to a paper towel lined plate to dry.

Step 6: Once everything is included, taste it to see on the off chance that you need to include more salt or pepper some time recently isolating into 4 bowls similarly. Beat with cheese, avocado, cilantro, fresh tortilla strips, lime juice, and jalapeño cuts

Chicken Chili Verde
Fixings & Substitutions
- Tomatillos husked and divided
- Poblano Peppers
- Anaheim Peppers
- Jalapeño Pepper

- Yellow Onion
- Garlic Cloves
- Cilantro
- Lime
- Ground Cumin
- Legitimate Salt
- Dark Pepper naturally ground
- Chicken Stock
- Chicken Thighs

How to Create Chicken Chili Verde

Stage 1: Put tomatillos cut side down, poblano peppers, anaheim peppers, jalapeños and unpeeled garlic cloves on a foil-lined enormous getting ready sheet. Put inside the grill on sear for 10 minutes or until the tomatillos and peppers scorch.

Step 2: Exchange the poblano and jalapeno peppers to a glass bowl and seal with plastic wrap to steam (take off the tomatillos and garlic on the preparing sheet for presently). After steaming for 10 minutes, evacuate skin and dispose of.

Step 3: In a blender, combine the tomatillos and all their juices, peeled garlic cloves, arranged broiled and peeled peppers, cilantro, lime juice, cumin, salt, pepper and chicken stock. Mix the fixings until they are well combined.

Step 4: Season chicken thighs with 1 teaspoon legitimate salt and 1 teaspoon ground dark peppe

Step 5: In a huge overwhelming foot skillet or dutch stove, include 2 tablespoon olive oil and warm over medium tall warm. Include the chicken and burn both sides until brilliant brown.

Step 6: Include the onions and saute for a couple of minutes some time recently including the blend from the blender.

Step 7: Include the verde blend. Bring the blend to a bubble, decrease warm to medium and cover and simmer for 20-30 minutes until the chicken is cooked through and shreds effectively with a fork.

Step 8: Taste and alter salt and pepper as required. Serve in a bowl with tortilla chips on the side and tons cilantro on beat.

Stacked Chicken Pho (Instant Pot + Stove Best)

You'll make this Stacked Chicken Pho within the Moment Pot, or on the stove beat – you're welcome. Either way it's getting to be stacked with all the treats, flavor, and you're attending to cherish it.

Fixings

For the Broth:
- 2 teaspoons olive oil
- 3 inch piece of ginger peeled and cut into huge pieces
- 1 yellow onion daintily cut
- 4 cloves of garlic skin evacuated
- 1 adhere lemongrass broken into huge pieces (discretionary)
- 4 mugs chicken stock or broth
- 1 star anise
- 2 tablespoons soy sauce
- 4 bone in chicken thighs
- 1 glass new cilantro
- 1 tablespoon coriander seeds
- 1 teaspoon black peppercorns

For the bowls:

- 5 ounces rice noodles
- 1 glass bean grows
- 4 scallions cut
- ¼ container new cilantro takes off picked off
- 1 jalapeño pepper meagerly cut
- Fresh mint takes off
- Fresh Thai basil takes off
- 2 limes cut
- Sriracha

Enlightening

For the Moment Pot

- Turn your weight cooker onto sauté and include the oil, onions and ginger. Cook for 4-5 minutes until beginning to caramelize. Blend within the broth, soy sauce, lemongrass, star anise, garlic, chicken thighs, cilantro, coriander seeds and peppercorn. Seal and cook on tall weight for 18 minutes. After 18 minutes, do the fast discharge and expel chicken to a clean surface. Strain the solids from the fluid and put the fluid back into the weight cooker.
- Turn the weight cooker to sauté and bring the broth to a bubble. Include the noodles and cook until done, almost 4 minutes.
- Whereas the noodles are cooking, evacuate the chicken from the bone and shred. Put break even with sums of the chicken into 4 bowls and best with the noodles and broth. Best with the bean grows, scallions, cilantro, cut jalapeño, mint, basil and lime juice.
- For the Stove Best
- Warm an overwhelming foot Dutch Broiler over medium tall warm and include the oil. Once hot, include the onions and ginger and sauté for 4-5 minutes until beginning to caramelize. Blend within the

broth, soy sauce, lemongrass, star anise, garlic, chicken thighs, cilantro, coriander seeds and peppercorn. Bring to a bubble and after that diminish to a stew, with the cover on, and cook for about 20 minutes until the chicken is completely cooked. Evacuate the chicken to a cutting board and strain the solids from the fluid and put the liquid back into the Dutch Stove.

- Turn the warm to medium tall and bring the broth to a bubble. Include the noodles and cook until done, approximately 4 minutes.
- Whereas the noodles are cooking, evacuate the chicken from the bone and shred. Put rise to sums of the chicken into 4 bowls and best with the noodles and broth. Best with the bean grows, scallions, cilantro, cut jalapeño, mint, basil and lime juice.

Smoky Chipotle Chicken Chili

A simple recipe for Chipotle Chicken Chili that's beyond any doubt to knock your socks off. Pile it tall with avocado, since duh, additionally cheese since that's obligatory!

Fixings
- 2 tablespoons olive oil
- 1 ruddy bell pepper generally chopped
- 1 orange or yellow chime pepper roughly chopped
- 1 poblano pepper generally chopped
- 1 yellow onion generally chopped
- 1 ruddy onion generally chopped
- 3 cloves garlic

- 2 tablespoons chili powder
- 1 pound ground chicken dim meat preferred
- 1-2 chipotle chilies (utilize 1 if you do not need as well much zest) finely chopped
- 2 tablespoons adobo sauce
- 1 ½ mugs smashed tomatoes
- 1 container chicken stock
- 1 16- ounce can of dark beans depleted and flushed
- Garnishes
- Shredded Cheddar Cheese Scallions, Diced Avocado, Acrid Cream, Cilantro or Chives

Enlightening

- In an expansive overwhelming foot pot, include the olive oil over medium tall warm.
- Include the ruddy and orange chime pepper, poblano pepper and yellow and ruddy onion and sauté for 10-12 minutes until the vegetables begin to cook down. Include the garlic and chili powder and sauté for 1-2 more minutes.
- Next, include the ground chicken. Break it up into pieces with a wooden spoon and sauté until brilliant brown.
- When the chicken is cooked, incorporate hacked chipotle bean stew peppers, adobo sauce, crushed tomatoes and chicken stock. Blend to combine and decrease the warm to medium. Include the drained black beans and stew for 20 minutes until the chili thickens.
- Once the chili has thickened, you'll diminish the warm to moo and keep it on the stove until you are prepared to serve.
- Best with any of the discretionary toppings and appreciate.

NOTES

Utilize all your favorite chili garnishes here. Acrid cream is idealize to cut the heat a bit.

Chicken Posole

The as it were kind of chicken soup that graces my kitchen may be a majorly flavorful Chicken Posole! It's past simple and puts your conventional chicken noodle soup to disgrace.

Fixings
- 1 pound chicken breast
- 4 mugs chicken stock
- 1 inlet leaf
- ½ teaspoon chopped new thyme
- ½ teaspoon chopped new oregano
- 2 clove garlic pulverized
- 1 teaspoon cumin
- 1 teaspoon salt
- ¾ teaspoon chili powder
- ½ teaspoon coriander
- ¼ teaspoon ruddy pepper drops
- 1 cup canned hominy drained and washed

Discretionary Fixings
- Diced avocado
- Lime wedges
- Chopped cilantro
- Crumbled cotija cheese
- Slivered Scallions

- Crema
- Tortilla Chips to serve on the side and scoop up anything within the bowl

Informational
- Exchange the chicken breasts onto a huge cutting board and carefully slice them in half so you have got thinly cut pieces. Sprinkle them on the two sides with salt and pepper.
- Warm a tablespoon of oil in a skillet over medium-high warm. Include the chicken breast in a single layer and burn for 1 minute on both sides until brilliant brown. Turn the warm to low, cover the pan, and cook for 12 minutes more, flipping the chicken midway to completely cook. Once cooked, set the chicken aside.
- Include the chicken broth to a medium Dutch stove and bring it to a fast stew. Once stewing, include the cove leaf, thyme, oregano, garlic, cumin, ½ teaspoon of the salt, chili powder, coriander, and ruddy pepper pieces. Diminish the warm to moo and stew for 15 minutes.
- Utilizing 2 forks, shred the chicken into little pieces. Add the chicken and depleted hominy to the Dutch oven. Raise the warm to medium to warm everything through. Taste and add more salt or other seasonings on the off chance that required. Dispose of the cove leaf.
- Serve the soup in person bowls with any of the specified garnishes.

NOTES

Make beyond any doubt you're employing a skillet that incorporates a well-fitting lid. This will keep your chicken from drying out whereas cooking through.

Simple Mexican Shredded Chicken

The most effortless Destroyed Chicken recipe that works for tacos, enchiladas, quesadillas etc.

Fixings
- 6 Boneless Skinless Chicken Thighs
- Kosher Salt and Naturally Split Dark Pepper
- 2 tablespoons Olive Oil
- 1 glass Chipotle Salsa or your favorite store bought salsa

Enlightening

For a moderate cooker (5-6 hours)
- Season the chicken thighs with salt and pepper on the two sides.
- Include the chicken into a moderate cooker beside the olive oil and salsa. Turn to tall warm and cook for 5-6 hours until the chicken is falling separated. Utilizing 2 forks, shred the chicken whereas still within the moderate cooker and let it rest within the salsa some time recently serving.

For a Dutch Oven (30 minutes)
- Season the chicken thighs with salt and pepper on the two sides.
- Put an expansive skillet with olive oil over tall warm and let the oil warm for a minute. Employing a pair of tongs, add the chicken to the skillet and sear the chicken on both sides for 3 minutes each so that each side is brilliant brown.
- Include the salsas to the skillet and cover the skillet with a tight fitting cover. Decrease the warm to medium and let the chicken cook for 25-30 minutes.
- After 20 minutes, utilizing a match of tongs, flip the chicken over to the over side and proceed to cook for another 10 minutes. Turn the heat off and utilizing 2 forks, shred the chicken and at that point utilize as required.

For an Moment Pot
- Season the chicken thighs with salt and pepper on both sides.
- Turn an moment pot onto the saute setting. Include the olive oil and let the oil warm for a minute. Employing a combine of tongs, include the chicken to the moment pot and burn the chicken on both sides for 3 minutes each so that each side is brilliant brown. Add the salsa on top, close the cover and make beyond any doubt it's sealed, and set the instant pot to poultry. Let the chicken cook and expel once the moment pot is done. Shred with 2 forks and serve as required.

Skillet Chipotle Chicken Enchilada Prepare
Fixings & Substitutions
- Boneless Skinless Chicken Breasts or thighs
- Enchilada Sauce
- Green Chiles
- Chipotles in adobo
- Monterey Jack Cheese destroyed
- Corn Tortillas
- Dark Beans
- New Corn expelled from the cob
- Scallions and Cilantro to decorate

How to Create Chipotle Chicken Enchilada Heat

Step 1: Combine the chicken, enchilada sauce, green chiles and chipotle peppers in an overwhelming foot pot over medium warm, mix everything to combine, and cook for 20 minutes until the chicken is cooked through.

Step 2: Expel the chicken, and utilizing 2 forks, shred the chicken. Save all of the sauce.

Step 3: Preheat the stove to 375 degrees F. In a medium measured skillet, layer the fixings, beginning with a layer of sauce taken after by 3 tortillas, ½ of the chicken, ½ of the dark beans, ½ of the corn, ½ of the cheese.

Step 4: Rehash for the moment layer with the remaining sauce, tortillas, chicken, dark beans, corn and cheese. Prepare for 20 to 30 minutes revealed, until bubbly and cheese has dissolved and begun to brown on beat.

Step 5: Beat with scallions and cilantro to serve. Cut into wedges as required.

Green Chicken Enchiladas
Fixings
- Rotisserie Chicken - hot tip shred the chicken in your blender to spare time whereas making these Green Chicken Enchiladas
- Flavors - I like to use ground coriander, ruddy pepper drops, and legitimate salt to season the chicken blend
- Vegetable Oil - safflower oil or avocado oil too works for warming the tortillas
- Flour Tortillas - you'll be able utilize corn tortillas, see my note on the substitution underneath

- Cheese - I utilize a blend of destroyed Monterey Jack cheese and cotija cheese
- Crema - we're whipping up a fast crema to sprinkle on best of our enchiladas utilizing crème fraîche and a sprinkle of drain
- Hand crafted Tomatillo Sauce - the recipe is underneath and super simple to create, everything beautiful much gets tossed into a blender
- Ruddy Onion and Cilantro - to decorate on beat of the Green Chicken Enchiladas

Varieties and Substitutions
- Green Enchilada Sauce – Whereas the homemade green enchilada sauce in this formula with shake your world you'll completely take a store-bought easy route and utilize your favorite jostled green enchilada sauce instep.
- Cheese – I adore a Montery Jack and Cotija cheese minute since it softens so delightfully. Cheddar, Colby Jack, Pepper Jack, a Mexican-blend or anything comparable would moreover work brilliantly!
- Flour Tortillas - Customarily enchiladas are made with corn tortillas, but you'll see that this formula calls for flour tortillas. Typically fair my individual inclination, I discover flour tortillas simpler to roll and less likely to break compared to corn tortillas. That being said, feel free to utilize corn tortillas in this formula.

How to Create Green Chicken Enchiladas

Step 1: Preheat the broiler to 425 degrees F. Sprinkle the olive oil over onion, poblano, and tomatillos on a preparing sheet and cook until vegetables are delicate and browned, 35–40 minutes. Let cool somewhat some time recently peeling the skin off the poblano.

Step 2: Exchange the blend and any juices to a blender. Include serrano chiles, garlic, chicken stock, cilantro, and lime juice and purée until smooth.

Step 3: Exchange to a large bowl, at that point season with salt and pepper as required.

Step 4: Include the chicken with the ground coriander, ruddy pepper chips, and ½ container green sauce in a huge bowl and season with salt and pepper.

Step 5: Hurl to combine.

Step 6: Warm vegetable oil in a medium skillet over medium-high. Working one at a time, fry the tortilla, turning once, almost 5 seconds per side. Exchange tortilla to paper towels to deplete. Rehash with remaining tortillas.

Step 7: Plunge both sides of each tortilla in green sauce just to coat, at that point exchange to a preparing sheet.

Step 8: Spread 1 glass green sauce longwise down the center of a 13×9" preparing dish. Working one at a time, spoon ¼ glass of the chicken blend into the center of the tortilla and crease one side over the filling, at that point proceed to roll the enchilada up like a burrito. Put crease side down within the arranged heating dish as you go, fitting them all in.

Step 9: Best with the remaining green sauce and after that heap on the cheese.

Step 10: Prepare until sauce is bubbling and cheese is starting to brown, 20–25 minutes.

Step 11: Whereas the enchiladas are preparing, combine the crème fraîche and drain and season with salt.

Step 12: Serve enchiladas topped with cheese, a sprinkle of crema, cut onion and cilantro.

DIY Chipotle Burrito Bowl
Chipotle Burrito Bowl Fixings
Ever wonder what is in a burrito bowl at Chipotle? Well here you go!
Variations and Subs
In case you're cooking for a gather that has distinctive dietary limitations or for picky eaters, this copycat chipotle chicken burrito bowls Is reaching to be your best companion. You'll be able serve the chicken, rice, and all garnishes independently and let everybody gather their bowls with anything they like. They are really one of my favorite simple supper thoughts that permits everybody to reproduce their go-to chipotle burrito bowl arrange from domestic!

For the Chicken
- Vegetable Oil
- Chipotle Peppers
- Garlic Powder
- Ground Cumin
- Dried Oregano
- Dark Pepper
- Legitimate Salt
- Boneless Skinless Chicken Thighs
- For the Rice
- Vegetable Oil
- White Basmati Rice
- Water
- Lime
- Chopped Cilantro
- Legitimate Salt

For the Garnishes

- Pinto Beans
- Solidified Charred Corn
- Guacamole
- Pico de Gallo
- Monterey Jack Cheese

How to Create a The Chipotle Burrito Bowl

Step 1: In an overwhelming pot, warm the oil over medium warm. Once hot, include the white rice and lime juice and sauté for 60 seconds to toast the rice.

Step 2: Add the water and bring the rice to a bubble. Cover and diminish the warm to moo and cook until the rice is delicate and all the water is retained.

Step 3: Once cooked add the cilantro and lighten the rice with a fork. Set aside and get begun on the chipotle chicken marinade.

Step 4: Combine the vegetable oil, chopped chipotle peppers in adobo, garlic powder, cumin, dried oregano, and dark pepper in a little bowl.

Step 5: Place the chicken in a huge zip best plastic pack and include the marinade. Zip the sack and blend the chicken into the marinade. Place it into the cooler and let it marinate for at slightest 1 hour.

Step 6: Flame broil the chicken 5 to 6 minutes per side, until the chicken is cooked. Expel the chicken from the flame broil and let rest for 10 minutes to bolt within the juices some time recently chopping.

Simple Taco Serving of mixed greens
Fixings & Substitutions
- Shallot

- Cilantro
- Garlic
- Ruddy Pepper Pieces
- Olive Oil
- Ruddy Wine Vinegar
- Salt
- Ground Turkey
- Yellow Onion
- Taco Flavoring
- Romaine Lettuce
- Cherry Tomatoes
- Cheddar Cheese
- Corn
- Avocados
- Green Onions
- Cilantro
- Black Beans

How to Create Taco Salad

Step 1: For the Cilantro Vinaigrette combine all the fixings in a blender and mix for 2 minutes until smooth. Taste and alter salt and pepper as required and set aside.

Step 2: For the taco meat put a medium skillet over medium tall heat and add the olive oil. Include the onions and sauté for 5 minutes until delicate.

Step 3: Include the garlic and sauté for 30 seconds more.

Step 4: Include the ground chicken or turkey and proceed to cook for 6-7 minutes until fully cooked. Include the taco flavoring and the water and decrease warm to moo. Stew the blend for 5 minutes whereas you amass the serving of mixed greens.

Step 5: In case you're layering this Taco Serving of mixed greens in one expansive serving bowl, layer half of the lettuce on the foot taken after by half of all the other garnishes.

Step 6: Add the following layer of lettuce on best and wrap up with the remaining toppings. Top with the meat and hurl along with some tablespoons of the vinaigrette. Include more as needed and serve instantly.

Ground Chicken Tacos
Fixings & Substitutions
Substitutions

Swap out the ground chicken in these Ground Chicken Tacos for ground hamburger or turkey in the event that you'd like.

While I've been making this formula and utilizing it in tacos for the past few months, you'll too make this ground chicken blend, discard the taco fixings, and utilize it as required. The same goes with any remains you might have from your DIY taco night. You'll put it into a rice/quinoa taco bowl. Utilize it in this southwestern lasagna. Toss it on best of your taco serving of mixed greens. Make chicken flautas. Skies the restrain.

Fixings

- Ground Chicken – You'll be able to substitute this for ground meat or turkey.
- Taco Flavoring – The key to making the most flavorful taco meat is my taco seasoning. I utilize it on almost EVERYTHING, simmering vegetables, seasoning refried beans, chili, you title it! Be that as it may, it is particularly scrumptious in these chicken tacos. This custom made zest blend employments spices we all probably have on hand and can be whipped up in under a few minutes.

- Tortillas – I'm obsessed with Vista Hermosa flour tortillas! I found them at Erewhon.
- Destroyed Cheese – I like utilizing a blend of naturally destroyed cheddar and naturally destroyed Monterey jack.
- Salsa – Utilize your favorite:
- ruddy, green, mellow, medium, or hot.
- Avocado or Guacamole – Ground Chicken Tacos would not be total without a little guac.

How to Create Ground Chicken Tacos

Step 1: Warm the olive oil in a large skillet over medium tall warm. Include the ground meat.

Step 2: Sauté the ground meat for 5 minutes and break it up with the back of a wooden spoon.

Step 3: Include all the taco flavoring and stir to combine.

Step 4: Proceed to cook the ground meat until it's fully cooked and no pink remains. Once cooked, include 2 tablespoons of water and decrease to a simmer. Let stew for 10 minutes.

Chicken Tinga Tacos

Destroyed chicken cooked within the most insane tasty spiced sauce on the planet and after that stuffed in a taco is supreme flawlessness.

INGREDIENTS

- 1 tablespoon olive oil
- 1 ½ pounds boneless skinless chicken thighs
- 1 yellow onion little dice
- 2 cloves garlic generally chopped
- 1 huge tomatillo husk expelled, flushed, and generally chopped

- ½ teaspoon oregano
- ¼ teaspoon ground cumin
- 1 14.5-ounce can fire-roasted tomatoes
- 2 tablespoons generally chopped chipotles additionally 2 tablespoons adobo sauce
- ½ container low-sodium chicken stock
- 1 narrows leaf
- Kosher salt

Garnishes
- Corn or flour tortillas
- Avocado diced
- 1 white onion diced
- Cilantro generally chopped
- Scallions cut
- Cotija disintegrated
- Lime wedges

Informational
- Warm oil in a Dutch stove or expansive pot over medium-high warm until gleaming. Include chicken thighs and cook until well browned, almost 6 minutes. Flip thighs and proceed to cook until other side is softly browned, around 3 minutes. Exchange chicken to a plate, clearing out fat in container, and set aside.
- Include onions and garlic to the same Dutch stove and cook, blending once in a while, until onions have browned around the edges, approximately 5 minutes. Add tomatillo and cook until browned around the edges, about 4 minutes. Include oregano and cumin and cook until fragrant, almost 30 seconds. Include tomatoes, chipotle, and adobo sauce and mix to combine. Evacuate from warm.

- Exchange sauce to a blender and puree until smooth. Pour sauce back into skillet, blend in chicken stock and inlet leaf, and bring to a bubble over medium warm. Settle chicken thighs in sauce, decrease to a stew, and cook until chicken is completely cooked and effortlessly destroyed, almost 15-20 minutes. Exchange chicken to a plate and let sit until cool sufficient to handle. Expel sauce from warm and dispose of narrows leaf.
- Drag chicken meat into strips. Mix chicken into sauce and cook over medium warm until warmed through, almost 3 minutes. Expel from warm and season with salt to taste.
- Warm the tortillas over an open fire to char, prep the white onion, avocado chopped cilantro, cut scallions, disintegrated cotija cheese, and lime wedges for serving
- Spoon chicken into warm tortillas and best with avocado, onion, cilantro, and cotija cheese. Serve with lime wedges.

NOTES

The avocado will differentiate pleasantly and tone down the flavors. You can also include acrid cream to your taco.

Chrissy's Chicken Nachos with Avocado Salsa
Fixings
- 1 8-ounce pack tortilla chips
- 2 mugs pulled chicken formula underneath
- 1 pound destroyed pepper Jack cheese also more as required

For the BBQ Pulled Chicken
- 1 ½ lbs boneless skinless chicken thighs

- kosher salt and crisply broken dark pepper
- 2 tablespoons olive oil
- 1 yellow onion meagerly cut
- 3 cloves garlic generally chopped
- 2 tablespoons tomato glue
- ½ container ketchup
- ⅓ glass tomato sauce
- ¼ container apple cider vinegar
- 2 tablespoons brown sugar
- 1 tablespoons finely chopped canned chipotle in adobo
- 1 teaspoon mustard powder

For the salsa:
- 2 expansive avocados diced
- 1 little ruddy onion finely diced
- 1 to mato diced
- 2 tablespoons chopped new cilantro
- Grated pizzazz and juice of 1 lime
- Kosher salt and naturally ground dark pepper

Garnishes
- Sour cream
- Sliced new or cured jalapeños
- Fresh cilantro

Informational
- Season the chicken with salt and pepper. In a medium dutch broiler, warm the oil over medium high warm until sparkling and hot. Include the chicken in one layer and brown until brilliant on both sides. Exchange to a plate and set aside.

- Include the onion to the dutch broiler and cook, blending every so often until brilliant, almost 9-10 minutes. Include the tomato glue and cook for 2 minutes. Include the ketchup, tomato sauce, ¼ glass water, vinegar, brown sugar, chipotles, mustard powder and season with salt and pepper. Bring to a bubble, diminish to a stew, and cook revealed until thick around 5 minutes.
- Return the chicken to the container and cover and stew for 1 hour until the chicken falls separated. Evacuate from the warm and cool. Shred the chicken with 2 forks.
- Preheat the broiler to 375°F.
- Organize the chips on a huge rimmed heating sheet in a single layer. Best with the pulled chicken and after that the pepper Jack cheese. Prepare until the cheese is bubbling and the edges of the chips are fresh, 20 to 25 minutes.
- In an expansive bowl, tenderly hurl together the avocados, onion, tomato, cilantro, lime get-up-and-go, lime juice, and salt and pepper to taste.
- Evacuate the nachos from the stove and top with the salsa, acrid cream, jalapeños, and cilantro.

NOTES

Everyone can eat off the sheet dish as a communal supper, or utilize tongs to plate them out and let everybody include their possess garnishes.

Poblano Chicken Fajitas
Fixings
- 1 poblano pepper meagerly cut
- 1 ruddy chime pepper daintily cut

- 1 yellow pepper meagerly cut
- ½ yellow onion daintily cut
- ½ ruddy onion daintily cut

For the Chicken
- 1 ½ lb chicken breasts
- 2 tablespoon lime juice
- 3 tablespoon olive oil
- 1 garlic clove minced
- ½ teaspoon salt
- ½ teaspoon ground cumin
- ½ teaspoon chili powder
- ½ teaspoon ruddy pepper chips

Enlightening
- Cut the chicken breasts into lean strips, almost the estimate of your finger. Combine the lime juice, olive oil, garlic, salt, cumin, chili powder and ruddy pepper chips in a bowl and whisk to combine. Include the chicken and marinate for 1 hour.
- Warm an expansive cast press skillet over tall warm. Include a tablespoon of olive oil. Include the chicken blend, marinade included, and sauté until completely cooked. Employing a pair of tongs, evacuate the chicken from the skillet and add the vegetables. Sauté until delicate and charred. Include the chicken back into the cast press skillet and hurl to combine.
- Serve nearby flour tortillas and best with wanted fixings such as avocado, acrid cream, guacamole and new lime juice.

NOTES

Expelling the seeds and films implies the poblano won't be as well zesty.

Enfrijoladas

Fixings & Substitutions

- Dark Beans
- Chipotles in Adobo
- Garlic
- Salt
- Water
- Corn Tortillas
- Onion finely chopped
- Monterey Jack Cheese destroyed
- Rotisserie Chicken destroyed
- Cilantro
- Crema
- Queso Fresco

How to Create Enfrijoladas

Step 1: Pre-heat broiler to 425 degrees F. Include the beans, garlic, chipotles and salt to a blender and puree until smooth.

Step 2: Include stock (or water) until the puree has the consistency of a thick soup.

Step 3: Exchange most of the blend to a huge shallow bowl and line a baking dish with approximately ⅓ container of the blend to make a base layer.

Step 4: Warm the corn tortillas marginally over a flame, or within the microwave. Plunge one side of a tortilla in the bean puree.

Step 5: Flip the tortilla and include a couple of tablespoons of onions, destroyed cheese and chicken. Roll the tortilla up and put in a preparing dish crease side down into the bean puree.

Step 6: Continue with the remaining tortillas and fillings. Cover the tortillas within the heating dish with the remaining bean puree and sprinkle with any remaining Monterey jack cheese.

Step 7: Heat for 8-10 minutes or until the cheese has liquefied. Serve instantly and beat with queso fresco, cilantro and crema.

Tacky Chicken Taco Chili Pasta

This Corny Chicken Taco Chili Pasta has taco flavors, tons of salsa, a few beans, and all the cheese.

Fixings
- 2 tablespoons olive oil
- 1 pound ground chicken
- 3 tablespoons taco flavoring
- 1 yellow onion chopped
- 6 cloves garlic chopped
- 1 ruddy chime pepper chopped
- 1 10- ounce can diced fire broiled tomatoes with green chiles
- 1 14- ounce can dark beans
- 1 8- ounce jolt chipotle salsa
- 1 glass refried beans
- 3 cups chicken broth
- 8 ounces pasta shells
- 1 container destroyed pepper jack cheese

- Fresh cilantro and green onions for garnish

Enlightening
- In a huge shallow finish skillet, warm the olive oil over medium tall warm. Include the chicken and break it up with the back of a wooden spoon whereas cooking until no pink remains. Include the taco seasoning to toast the flavors and blend to combine. Include onion, garlic, and chime pepper. Mix to combine and cook for 5 minutes. Include tomatoes, beans, salsa and Swanson Chicken Broth. Bring to a bubble, diminish to a stew for 15 minutes.
- Stir within the pasta and stew, until pasta is cooked through.
- Evacuate pot from warm, sprinkle the cheese on beat (permit to soften in the event that craved) and decorate with herbs

Zuni Simmered Entire Chicken with Chimichurri

The leading Simmered Entirety Chicken with an idiot proof strategy for the most fresh skin!

Fixings

For the Chicken:
- 1 4-5 pound entire chicken giblets removed
- 3 tablespoons legitimate salt
- ¼ teaspoon naturally cracked black pepper
- 2 tablespoons blended herbs, like thyme, rosemary, and sage finely chopped
- 2 tablespoons additional virgin olive oil

For the Chimichurri:

- 1 head parsley
- 1 head cilantro
- 20 takes off basil
- 2 cloves garlic
- 2 tablespoons capers flushed
- 2 tablespoons ruddy wine vinegar
- ½ - ¾ container olive oil
- kosher salt and naturally split dark pepper to taste

Informational

For the Chimichurri:

- In a nourishment processor, combine herbs, garlic, and vinegar and capers. Beat until coarsely chopped, 20-40 seconds. Exchange to a small bowl and mix in olive oil. Season with salt and pepper.
- For the Chicken:
- Dry brine for the chicken begins 24-48 hours ahead of serving. Begin by tapping the chicken all over with paper towels to create beyond any doubt its exceptionally dry. Utilize your fingers to release the skin on the breast making a pocket that you'll utilize to put the chopped herbs.
- Put the chicken onto a rack in a simmering dish and sprinkle generously with the salt making beyond any doubt to get the bottom, inside depth wings. Tuck the wings behind the breast and tie the legs. Gently sprinkle with pepper Put chicken revealed into the refrigerator for 24-48 hours, this will gradually get dried out the skin, the conclusion result after broiling will be the foremost fresh skin ever.
- After the chicken has discuss dried, expel from the fridge, and let sit at room temp for almost 30 min whereas the broiler preheated to

425. Stuff the herbs into the opening you cut the day earlier. Sprinkle the chicken with 2 tablespoons olive oil and broil within the preheated stove for 1 hour, 15 min, turn the feathered creature ½ way to guarantee indeed browning. Once done, a meat thermometer ought to enlist at 165 degrees F and the juices ought to run clean. Expel from the broiler and let rest 10-15 minutes before carving.

Flame broiled Lemonade Chicken
This Barbecued Lemonade Chicken is the culminate summer fundamental course. The lemonade-based marinade is the mystery to super flavorful barbecued chicken and a pleasant brilliant hull.
Fixings
- 8 little bone-in, skin-on chicken leg quarters
- 4 glasses Florida Natural® Lemonade
- 4 cloves garlic finely ground
- ¼ container Dijon mustard
- 2 tablespoons dried oregano
- 2 tablespoons granulated onion powder
- 2 teaspoons ground cumin
- Kosher salt and naturally ground dark pepper
- Oil for the flame broil
- 3 expansive lemons

Enlightening
- Put the chicken in a huge zip beat sack. Whisk together the lemonade, garlic, mustard, oregano, dried onion, cumin, 1 tablespoon salt, and crisply broken dark pepper in a huge fluid

measuring container until combined. Pour over the chicken, making beyond any doubt all the pieces are secured and evacuate any overabundance discuss from the sack some time recently fixing. Exchange to a cooler and let marinate for 4 - 24 hours.

- Get ready a barbecue for medium warm, and softly oil the barbecue grates.
- Evacuate the chicken from the marinade. Save 2 mugs of marinade and dispose of the rest. Put the chicken on a paper towel-lined heating sheet and pat dry. Season the chicken generously with salt and pepper and organize the pieces skin-side down on the flame broil, taking off a few space between each. Cook until the skin is gently charred and discharges effectively from the barbecue, approximately 2 minutes. Turn the chicken pieces around 90 degrees so the skin won't burn and cook another 2 minutes. Flip the chicken skin-side up. Cover the flame broil and cook until an instant-read thermometer embedded into the thickest portion of each thigh peruses 165 degrees F, 20 to 25 minutes more. Exchange to a platter and let rest for approximately 5 minutes some time recently serving.
- In the meantime, exchange the saved marinade to a little non-stick pan and put on the hot flame broil or on a burner interior. Bring to a bubble, at that point proceed to cook until it has thickened somewhat and diminished by half, around 15-20 minutes.
- Pizzazz and juice one of the lemons and mix into the sauce. Exchange to a little bowl for serving. Cut the remaining 2 lemons in half crosswise.
- Put the lemon parts on the flame broil, flesh-side down, and barbecue until softly charred, 1 to 2 minutes. Serve nearby the chicken and sauce.

NOTES

Utilize this marinade on any cut of chicken. Fair be beyond any doubt to alter your cooking time and utilize a thermometer to check for doneness.

Lemon Broiled Spatchcock Chicken
Fixings & Substitutions
- Entirety Chicken
- Olive Oil additionally more for potatoes
- Dried Oregano
- Dried Thyme
- Lemon juiced and zested
- Chopped Rosemary
- Legitimate Salt and Dark Pepper crisply ground
- Garlic cut in half
- Lemons divided
- Child Potatoes

How to Form Simmered Spatchcock Chicken
Step 1: Begin by cutting along one side of the spine.
Step 2: Cut all the way to the beat and after that cut the other side of the spine. Evacuate the bone completely.
Step 3: Flip the chicken over and thrust it down together with your hand breaking the breast bone.
Step 4: Season with salt, pepper and herbs.
Step 5: Tuck lemons around the fowl for additional flavor.
Step 6: Include a few infant potatoes to splash up all the drippings.
Step 7: Sprinkle a few olive oil.

Step 8: Cook until the feathered creature is 165 degrees F.

Step 9: Evacuate and let rest for 15 minutes some time recently cutting and serving.

Chicken Larb Bowls
Fixings
For the speedy pickles:
- 2 Persian cucumbers meagerly cut
- ½ ruddy onion meagerly cut
- 2 tablespoons rice vinegar

For the chicken:
- 1 tablespoon vegetable oil
- 5 ounces kale deveined and chopped
- 1 pound ground chicken
- 2 cloves garlic finely chopped
- 6 scallions white and light green parts, daintily cut
- 2 to 3 tablespoons soy sauce
- 1 to 2 tablespoons sambal oelek
- 1 tablespoon brown sugar

For the rice:
- 2 glasses water
- 1 container coconut drain
- 1 teaspoon sugar
- 1 teaspoon legitimate salt
- 2 glasses jasmine rice
- zest and juice of 1 lime

- ***To decorate:***
- fresh mint takes off
- fresh basil clears out
- fresh cilantro clears out

Informational

To create the fast pickles:
- In a little bowl, hurl the cucumbers, ruddy onion, and vinegar. Set aside to marinate whereas you cook the chicken.

To make the chicken:
- In an expansive, heavy-bottomed skillet, warm the oil over medium-high warm. Include the kale and cook until shriveled, 5 to 6 minutes. Season with salt and carefully exchange to a medium bowl.
- Include the ground chicken to the same skillet and cook, breaking it separated with the back of a wooden spoon and mixing regularly until no pink remains, 8 to 10 minutes.
- Include the garlic and scallions and cook for 1 minute, or until fragrant. Include the soy sauce, sambal oelek, and brown sugar and blend to combine. Return the cooked kale to the skillet and mix to combine. Season with salt and diminish the warm to moo until prepared to serve.

To form the rice:
- Combine the water, coconut milk, sugar, and salt in a medium pan and warm over medium-high warm until the blend begins to stew. Include the rice and bring back to a low stew. Cover the pot, diminish the warm to moo, and cook undisturbed for almost 15 minutes, until all the fluid has been ingested.
- Turn off the warm and let the rice steam for another 5 to 10 minutes, until completely cooked and delicate. Reveal, cushion, and hurl within the lime pizzazz and juice.

To collect:
- Partition the rice among 4 bowls, taken after by the chicken and kale, pickles, and bounty of new mint, basil, and cilantro. Serve promptly.

Chicken Kofta Kebabs
Fixings
For the Kefta
- 1 medium zucchini
- 1 pound ground chicken white or dim meat
- ⅓ container cut scallions
- ⅓ cup chopped mint
- 3 tablespoons chopped cilantro
- 3 cloves garlic finely chopped
- 1 teaspoon ground cumin
- 1 teaspoon ground coriander
- 1 ½ teaspoon salt
- 2 tablespoons tahini
- 12 little wooden sticks drenched in water for 20 minutes

For the Sumac Dressing
- 4 teaspoons ground sumac doused in 4 teaspoons warm water for 15 minutes
- 3 tablespoons new lemon juice
- 2 tablespoons pomegranate molasses
- 2 cloves garlic minced
- 2 teaspoons ruddy wine vinegar

- ½ glass extra-virgin olive oil
- Kosher salt to taste

To Serve
- Tzatziki
- Pita Bread
- Pickled Ruddy Onions
- Hummus
- Charred Jalapeños

Enlightening

For the Kefta
- Grind zucchini, combine with ½ teaspoon salt and let sit for 5 minutes. Crush out as much fluid as conceivable. Blend together zucchini and remaining fixings in an expansive bowl. Partition the blend into 12 pieces, then with damp hands, shape around 12 splashed sticks.
- Warm a flame broil or grill container to medium tall, brush the kebabs with a bit of oil, then grill for 8-10 minutes on each side, or until cooked through.

For the Dressing
- In another littler bowl, water with splashed sumac, lemon juice, pomegranate molasses, garlic, ruddy wine vinegar and olive oil. Whisk to combine and season with salt as required.
- Sprinkle the dressing on beat of the chicken and serve with all the accouterments.

NOTES

No sticks, no issue! Instep, shape the kofta blend into patties and flame broil.

129

www.ingramcontent.com/pod-product-compliance
Lightning Source LLC
Chambersburg PA
CBHW062107220526
45471CB00010B/3639